# Foundations for Operating Department Practice

This book is due for return on or before the last date

# Foundations for Operating Department Practice

## Essential Theory for Practice

Edited by Hannah Abbott
and Helen Booth

Open University Press

Open University Press
McGraw-Hill Education
McGraw-Hill House
Shoppenhangers Road
Maidenhead
Berkshire
England
SL6 2QL

email: enquiries@openup.co.uk
world wide web: www.openup.co.uk

and Two Penn Plaza, New York, NY 10121-2289, USA

First published 2014

A catalogue record of this book is available from the British Library

ISBN-13: 978-0-33-524497-3 (pb)
eISBN: 978-0-33-524498-0

*Library of Congress Cataloging-in-Publication Data*
CIP data applied for

Typesetting and e-book compilations by
RefineCatch Limited, Bungay, Suffolk

Fictitious names of companies, products, people, characters and/or data that may be used herein (in case studies or in examples) are not intended to represent any real individual, company, product or event.

**Praise for this book**

"This book identifies strongly the enhanced development of the operating department practice (ODP) profession. It focuses well on the theory underpinning the need for the compassionate care of the patient. Compassionate care is a fundamental requirement of ODPs now, given the changes in the profession. Many years ago, the main role of the ODP was to give technical support to anaesthetists. This has completely changed and the focus is now on ensuring safe and effective perioperative patient care using enhanced and improved knowledge and skills. It is a fundamental requirement for ODPs to develop these advanced skills and knowledge in order to firmly establish the profession.

This book does not focus on clinical skills, it focuses on the role of the ODP in every-day work. This involves elements such as interprofessional working, research, patient safety, psychological aspects of patient care, and legal frameworks. Most ODP text books have not emphasised the importance of these topics – whereas this book does. The value of this book is firstly to emphasise the knowledge and understanding needed by ODPS to care for patients appropriately, and secondly, to emphasise the improvements that the profession has been undergoing over the past few years.

Based on the information within this book, students, practitioners, theatre managers and even surgeons and anaesthetists will be able to better understand the modern role of the ODP. Technical skills are obviously still important, but even more important is the safety and compassionate care of patients in the operating environment. This can only be achieved by a combination of knowledge and skills, working in harmony with other professionals.

This book will provide a sound basis for the promotion of the ODP profession and the better understanding of all other professionals on the way that ODPs now work."

Paul Wicker, Head of Perioperative Studies, Edge Hill University, Ormskirk, UK

# Contents

# List of contributors

**Hannah Abbott** (Editor) MSc (Science) (Open), PGCE, BSc (Hons), ODP, MCODP, FCODP, MIfL QTLS
Associate Head of School, School of Allied and Public Health Professions, Birmingham City University

**Helen Booth** (Editor) MA (Bioethics), BSc (Hons), Cert Ed, ODP, MCODP, FCODP
Chair of the Professional Council, College of Operating Department Practitioners

**Michael Donnellon** MBA, MA (Ed), PG Cert, FHEA, ODP, MCODP
Course Leader BSc (Hons) in Operating Department Practice, University of Central Lancashire

**Andrew Gulley** BSc (Hons) FHEA, ODP, MCODP
Deputy Head of Operating Department Practice, University of Leicester

**Penny Joyce** Ed D, M.Ed, BA Ed, FHEA, ODP, MCODP
Professional Practice Lead, School of Health Sciences and Social Work, University of Portsmouth

**Christine Mahoney** BSc (Hons), PGCE, ODP, MCODP
Senior Lecturer and Course Director (Perioperative Programmes), Faculty of Health and Social Care, London South Bank University

**Susan Parker** MA (Ed), BSc (Open), ODP, MCODP
Senior ODP Education and Quality Lead, University Hospital North Staffordshire

**Keith Underwood** ODP, MCODP, FCODP, Dip ICM
Lead Medical Devices Training Coordinator, York Teaching Hospital NHS Foundation Trust (Based at Scarborough Hospital)

**Stephen Wordsworth** Ed D, MSc (Health Care Practice), PG Cert, BA (Hons), Cert Ed, ODP, MCODP, FCODP
Head of School, School of Allied and Public Health Professions, Birmingham City University

# Foreword: the development of the Operating Department Practitioner

I am proud to write the foreword to this important book, specifically targeted at members of the profession of Operating Department Practitioner (ODP), written by ODPs for ODPs. This marks a milestone in the ongoing professional development of the ODP in that this book is the first to address specifically those aspects of the ODPs professional life and practice not covered in more generic clinical or technical texts.

It may be of interest to readers to speak a little about the history of our profession and the forces that helped to shape the profession of today. A helpful starting point is perhaps that first book written specifically for our profession. In contrast to the book that you are holding now the first book was written by two consultant anaesthetists at St. Thomas's Hospital in London, Dr Charles Foster and Dr Bridget Jepson. First published in 1968, its title *Anaesthesia for Operating Theatre Technicians* highlights the title adopted by the profession for the first 25–30 years of its organized existence.

The history of the profession can in fact be traced back to the eighteenth century, to a time that was not only before the advent of anaesthesia but also predates organized operating theatres, when surgery was carried out in general wards or even the home. But 1945 is the generally accepted date for the founding of the organized profession, when the College of Operating Department Practitioners was founded as the Association of Operating Theatre Technicians. This was driven in part by the renowned pioneer in anaesthesia, Sir Ivan Magill, who wished to see those men with whom he worked (and in those days it was exclusively men), become organized so as to promote common standards through organized training. The first formal training school was founded in 1947 at St. Thomas's Hospital in London and the nascent predecessor to the College established the first qualification in 1951, the Diploma. That year also saw the first of several name changes – to the Institute of Operating Theatre Technicians, thus the Diploma of the IOTT.

Fast forward to 1970 when the then Department of Health and Social Security commissioned a report on the Organization and Staffing of Operating Theatres, commonly known as the Lewin Report, after the Chair of the committee. For ODPs Lewin made two key recommendations, first, that the group then known as Theatre Technicians should in future be known as Operating Department Assistants (ODAs); and, second, that they should have a recognized career structure, with a common scheme of training and structured opportunities for progression to the role of Senior Operating Department Assistant. The first formal training centres were established in 1974 and the first national examinations were held in 1976. It is notable that these early examinations drew heavily from the question bank of the Association's Diploma examinations.

The next significant milestone and an early indication of the emergent professional status was the transfer of ODAs from the NHS staffs ancillary group to the Professional and Technical Group in 1983, following several years of lobbying by the College. The ancillary body was responsible for the terms and conditions of staff that we would now recognize as members of the estates, facilities and housekeeping teams.

In 1989 the NHS Executive, concerned about chronic staffing shortages and the cost of running operating theatres, commissioned the report, the Management and Utilization of Operating Theatres, better known as the Bevan Report. Bevan was the first official report to recommend that ODPs should become a regulated profession, something not ultimately achieved until 2004 after the College successfully lobbied both Parliament and the Health Professions Council (now the Health and Care Professions Council). Leading up to this the College maintained a voluntary register with codes of conduct and disciplinary processes. ODPs that transferred from the voluntary register held by the College to the statutory register within the HPC found that their College registration number transferred with them. This development of the profession has been exemplified by the development of our training and education; from the very first IOTT diploma, through the City and Guilds, National and Scottish Vocational Qualifications in the 1990s, the Higher Education Diploma to the new BSc Honours Degree in Operating Department Practice.

The first book written for the profession over 45 years ago opens with 'A GOOD technician learns his duties by practical work in the anaesthetic room and operating theatre' (Foster and Jepson, 1968: 1). This foundation of clinical practice remains essential for the ODP of today; however, this book reflects the fundamental principles that underpins the role of a Registered Practitioner. This includes the legal and ethical framework that governs our professional practice; reflection, research and learning in the perioperative environment that informs our practice; our role as part of the perioperative team and crucially the human factors and non-technical skills that are essential for ensuring patient safety.

Although our knowledge and understanding of team dynamics and what contributes to a safe clinical environment has developed beyond the recognition of those technician pioneers of our profession, our focus as practitioners is surely the same. It is therefore fitting that in commending this book to the modern operating department practitioner, I end with another passage from the professions' first book all those years ago.

The patient is the most important person in the anaesthetic room and operating theatre, and should be treated with respect in both thought and deed. The technician must bear this in mind at all times. The unconscious patient is at the mercy of everyone in the theatre and cannot protest.

(Foster and Jepson, 1968: 1)
Bill Kilvington ODP, FCODP, MCODP
President, The College of Operating Department Practitioners

## Reference:

Foster C. and Jepson B. (1968) *Anaesthesia for Operating Theatre Technicians*, London: Lloyd-Luke.

# Preface

This book has been written to support pre- and post-registration Operating Department Practitioners (ODPs) both during their undergraduate studies and throughout their professional careers. It has been written by ODPs from academic and clinical settings throughout the UK and, while the content may be relevant to other professionals, it is designed to meet the specific needs of the ODP profession.

As you will have read in the forward, the ODP profession has undergone a rapid development over the last 30 years; it is important to note that for a profession to establish itself as an independent profession with a unique body of knowledge in this short time is a remarkable achievement. While our clinical knowledge and skills have developed, this is not the most significant marker of the development of the profession; rather, it is the professional qualities, attributes, commitment to evidence-based care and an understanding of the wider context of care that qualifies us as registered practitioners in our own right. In recognition of these developments and to support the transition to an all-graduate profession, it was timely to write a book that encapsulates the professional skills and attributes in the unique context of the ODP profession.

This text does not include clinical skills as there are a number of existing texts that address these and, in addition, the dynamic nature of the environment means that journal articles are the best sources to ensure ODPs' clinical skills reflect the current evidence. The focus of this text is therefore the fundamental professional knowledge and skills which enable ODPs to deliver effective, compassionate and evidence-based care to the patient, and the continual development of this professional knowledge and skills. Each chapter explores the underpinning principles of the topic area, and then links this to practice with a clear focus on the application of knowledge through practice-based examples and 'stop and think' boxes to help you relate the principles to your own practice. This text provides you with information but we also hope it will act as a catalyst to encourage you to question practice and to undertake further reading in the subject areas included within the book.

While this book includes a number of distinctly different topics, you will find that a number of links can be made between them and these have been identified in each chapter. You will also find that the authors have written their chapters in slightly different styles. As editors we have welcomed this as we feel it is important that each chapter uses the language most suited to the given topic, and in addition we wanted to show that there are a number of different approaches to written work and hence would encourage you to develop your own style of academic/professional writing.

This book seeks to provide you with a good overview of fundamental topics; however, you should remember that these topic areas are extensive and therefore wider reading is important to develop your knowledge. You will find that each chapter is supported by evidence and there is a reference list at the back of each chapter that will serve as a good starting point for your wider reading. The evidence supporting the chapters within this book is drawn from contemporary and classical sources that reflect the context in which the knowledge was developed.

We hope that you will enjoy this book and find it helpful as you develop your career in this exciting and dynamic profession.

Hannah Abbott and Helen Booth

# Acknowledgements

We would like to thank Deborah Robinson for her contribution to this project, especially during the early stages of this work.

We would also like to acknowledge the College of Operating Department Practitioners for their support throughout this project.

Hannah Abbott and Helen Booth

# 1  Working in the perioperative team

## Hannah Abbott and Helen Booth

---

**Key topics**

- Development of teams
- The individual Operating Department Practioner (ODP) within the team

- Communication for effective teamworking
- Clinical supervision

---

## Introduction

The complexity of working within the perioperative environment requires the ODP, who works alongside a wide variety of different professionals, to have highly developed communication and teamworking skills. In addition to communication and teamworking skills the ODP needs to have developed a skill set that allows them to manage the range of complex and often stressful situations that present in the perioperative environment. This chapter therefore aims to explore the knowledge and skills that the ODP needs to develop to work within the team and as an individual within the team.

While communications and teamworking are vast subjects, this chapter reviews some of the key concepts involved and, hopefully, will also inspire you to read more about those of particular interest. The perioperative team is a team of professionals who have developed their knowledge and skills to deliver safe, effective and evidence-based care to the perioperative patient. Many of the concepts explored in this chapter therefore also relate to discussions in other chapters within this book. This is not repetition for its own sake but rather an indication of how important these topics are to many different aspects of operating department practice and how the fundamental knowledge explored in this text is integral to the care delivered by the perioperative team.

## Why is this relevant?

The perioperative environment is a challenging and potentially high-risk environment where a number of different healthcare practitioners work together to deliver high-quality care to the patient. In order to deliver this care, it is therefore essential that the ODP is 'able to work appropriately with others' (Health and Care Professions Council (HCPC), 2014, Standard 9) and must be able to understand the importance of building and maintaining professional relationships as both an individual practitioner and collaboratively as a member of a team (HCPC, 2014). The inclusion of teamworking within both the threshold standards for all ODPs and within the professional body (College of Operating Department Practitioners, CODP) pre-registration curriculum demonstrates the fundamental need for all ODPs to be able to work effectively within the perioperative team and hence within the perioperative environment.

## Teamworking

The crucial nature of teamworking in the perioperative environment has already been identified in this chapter but what do we mean when we use the phrase 'teamworking'? This is a commonly used phrase and many ODPs will have cited their ability to work in a team when applying to study operating department practice at university or when applying for jobs; in the same way many people will comment that 'he or she is not a team player', but what does this really mean?

There are a number of different definitions of a team; however, all of these have some shared characteristics. Teams are groups of people who work together or co-ordinate their actions to achieve a common goal. The perioperative team is known as a 'multidisciplinary' team that means it is comprised of individuals with a diverse range of professional backgrounds and this multidisciplinary nature has been shown to improve effectiveness and innovation in patient care (Borill et al., 2001). If you reflect on teams you may have been a member of in the past, you will probably consider that this definition will fit most teams. However, it is also important to think about how teams develop. Many people will have been part of teams in which they have taken an active role in forming; for example, when a group of individuals decide to participate in a team event together, and will have also been placed into an established team, for example, when starting a new job. Effective teams can be established in both ways; however, it is important for the ODP to understand how the team develops.

Teams within the perioperative environment tend to be dynamic and shift patterns dictate that there will be variation in the team members for any different day or different list, consequently the ODP may be involved in team development on a regular basis. A team always has to change to accommodate new members, irrespective of how established the team is and hence there will always be a period of adjustment for all team members when there is a change to the team. Although every team will develop in their own way, an exploration of teamworking concepts in a number of studies allowed Tuckman (1965) to propose a model of team development. Tuckman proposed that the team need to initially orient themselves by testing the boundaries and this is known as the 'forming' phase. Once a team is formed, it is inevitable that, as members start to work with each other, there will be some tensions and conflict. This is known as 'storming'; once this is resolved however the team will undergo a period of 'norming' where they develop their own standards and roles. The final stage in team development is 'performing' where the structure supports performance and the team are able to focus their energy on the task. This model illustrates that all teams have to undergo development and hence the ODP should be prepared for this when working within a new team; it is important to note that it is not a failing of the team if there are some challenges as the team develops but it is crucial that these are managed in a professional manner.

### Motivation and shared goals

Shared goals have been recognized as one of the defining characteristics of teams and the team then works together to achieve these shared goals (Health Care Development Agency, 2003). The achievement of these shared goals may therefore be considered to provide the key motivational driver for the team in working together effectively to achieve the goal. This is particularly true in the perioperative team where the overarching goal is related to the care of the patient and there is the professional expectation that all team members work towards this. This may be considered a direct contrast to some other teams that you may have experienced where there is an element of competition within the team.

Goal setting is an important part of teamworking; it is not possible to work together effectively unless all members of the team know what they are working towards. It is often assumed that that the perioperative team will have the shared goal of delivering a high standard of care and ensuring patient safety is optimized and, while this will be true for every case, this is a fairly generic goal and some cases will benefit from the identification of more specific goals. It is therefore essential that, as part of the team briefing, goals are identified for individual cases – these goals will be those that are required to achieve the overarching goal of safe, high-quality care. For example, in some cases, the priority may be to reduce the overall anaesthetic time. The entire team need to be aware of this to ensure that any delays on the surgical side are minimized, or alternatively the goal may be to avoid the need for blood transfusion and the whole team will need to be aware of the plans to reduce blood loss.

### Theatre etiquette/team culture

There is an established etiquette to working in the perioperative environment, and although this may vary slightly between hospitals there are a number of common themes (Box 1.1) that are essential for the new team member. The elements in Box 1.1 are indicative and there may be additions for specific theatres; however, those listed are common and therefore should be observed by any new individual within the perioperative team. As individuals become more familiar with a team, they will become aware of, and embedded in, the unique culture of the team and while this is generally welcomed by the individual, they must be careful that this does not impact adversely upon their professionalism, for example, by becoming overfamiliar in the professional environment.

---

**Box 1.1 Key elements of theatre etiquette**

- Practitioners should always be referred to by their title, until that individual tells you otherwise; for example Dr Jones (anaesthetist), Mrs Smith (Consultant Surgeon), Nurse, Charge Nurse or Sister (depending on grade); fellow ODPs may use either Mrs/Mr/Miss/Ms or ODP as their title.
- In front of patients, practitioners are always referred to by their title, irrespective of what the team would otherwise call them.
- At induction of anaesthesia, the theatre team should be silent; this means no audible activity as well as no verbal discussion.
- The accepted line of communication to the operating team is via the scrub practitioner as they will be able to determine whether it is an appropriate time in the surgery for the team to receive information.
- The theatre team should be generally quiet and should refrain from any personal discussions during surgery.
- There should be no distractions during the swab, needle and instrument counts.
- Practitioners historically remain standing during surgery, and while a number of theatres now allow the team to sit as appropriate, it would be advisable for new entrants to the perioperative team to remain standing until invited to sit.

---

Irrespective of whether ODPs are established members of a team or a new entrant, it is important that they recognize how the culture of the team may be perceived by others. The culture of a team that has been established for a long time with few changes of staff may act as a barrier to a new team member. This has the potential to result in a risk to the patient if the new team member feels that their contributions are unwelcome or they do not feel able to raise a concern. Equally, well-established teams may have developed their own team language, for example, by calling instruments/equipment by different names, and this can be confusing for other practitioners. It is therefore essential that teams recognize the culture they have established and support new team members in orientating to the team; in the same way new team members need to understand the importance of asking when unsure as this will expedite their integration into the team.

## The individual ODP within the team

One of the defining characteristics of a team is that they have their own identity and can therefore be recognized as a team by others (Health Care Development Agency, 2003). In the perioperative environment there are a number of teams: the big 'perioperative department team'; teams related to specific theatres; teams related to specific roles (e.g. the 'anaesthetic team'); or indeed teams related to specific shifts (e.g. the 'late' team). Many members of staff will belong to a number of these teams (e.g. the anaesthetic team and the vascular theatre team) while other teams will be more dynamic; for example, those linked to specific shifts. ODPs will also need to work alongside other teams who may come into theatre and also need to be able to work as a new, temporary, team member in other departments, for example, when the ODP is required in the emergency department or imaging department.

The ODP therefore needs to be able to work as an individual within a number of teams and to be able to integrate themselves within a 'new' team on a regular basis. In order to do this effectively the ODP needs to be able to recognize the value of the following.

### Confidence/assertiveness

Being confident for the ODP is not only about their knowledge and skill base; it is also an essential aspect of working within and with teams. A lack of self-confidence will affect the ODP's coping strategies when facing the challenges and problems that arise in operating theatres and related care areas. The lack of coping reinforces the lack of self-confidence resulting in a spiralling effect that can have an impact on how the practitioner works within a team. The obligation for the ODP to 'speak up' in the case of poor care being delivered has never been so prominent in the clinical environment and was identified as one of the key aspects of the Safe Surgery campaign.

There is a real need for the creation of a supportive environment, as this will contribute to the ODP's confidence, therefore enabling them to be assertive and to manage any issues effectively. Being able to manage situations well requires assertiveness, which is about being able to express yourself and to speak up, not only for your rights but that of the patients and others. Being assertive is not about challenging and seeking to dominate or belittle another individual, but is more about striving to improve, develop and deal with matters as they arise effectively.

It can be difficult to articulate concerns or opinions however, and timely communication is paramount in the acute setting of the operating theatre, but to not speak up is negating the ODP's responsibility and can condone the observed unacceptable behaviour. Using appropriate skills the ODP can carefully handle a situation to ensure a safety aspect is addressed, behaviour is moderated and others within the team meet and develop compliance with the expected standards.

### Knowledge base and personal experiences

Every perioperative team is comprised of a number of different professionals, each with their own specific professional knowledge and this will be reflected in the roles undertaken by each individual; these differentiated but defined roles are another characteristic of a team (Health Care Development Agency, 2003). It is therefore crucial that the ODP recognizes the specific knowledge that they contribute to the team and how this complements that of their colleagues. It should be remembered that it is not just the knowledge that may vary between professionals, but also the underpinning philosophy that governs how that knowledge is delivered; for example, there are differences between a 'medical model' of education and a 'nursing model'. The integration of interprofessional education in both pre- and post-registration education has aimed to embed the understanding of other professions with the intention of improving care delivery and teamworking; the ODP therefore should seek to maximize these learning opportunities. In order to work effectively within the team, the ODP needs to recognize the value of their own knowledge and be able to confidently assert this while recognizing the value of others' inputs.

Knowledge however is not purely formed from education, and personal experiences can impact how a practitioner may engage with the team regarding a specific case or issue. As we will explore further in the context of evidence-based practice, personal clinical experiences can make a significant contribution to the formation of professional knowledge. Here, however, is an important distinction, the difference between the professional experiences that as an ODP can inform our practice and the personal experiences, which we have to acknowledge and be able to 'set aside'. Personal experiences can have a profound influence on how we perceive a situation and so may hamper how a team decision-making process is viewed. The ODP should therefore be aware of this and be able to moderate it accordingly. In the same way, an ODP who has experienced a case as a patient may feel that their 'service user' view will help the team in delivering care to the patient. However, they need to consider whether it is professional to share this potentially sensitive information within a team. The ODP must ensure that their interactions within the team, while potentially friendly, must also be professional and sharing information that is personal is both unprofessional and can make other team members very uncomfortable thus adversely impacting the team dynamic.

## Clinical supervision

The fundamental desire of any ODP is to ensure that they improve and develop their practice through research, reflection and active participation in their learning. Clinical supervision can therefore support this professional development and the ODP who embraces supervision of their practice will see it as another tool of lifelong learning and an invaluable way to demonstrate their professional responsibility and accountability. Supervision may take a variety of forms, for example, managerially, clinically or professionally, but, the essence of the concept is to look at reviewing performance, discussion of cases, objectives or looking at development. Supervision also sets out training needs, modification of practice or levels of compliance with professional conduct and codes. The focus for the majority of ODPs will be clinical supervision as this addresses both the professional and personal aspect for those working in the perioperative environment, although the other forms of supervision may impact on the overall outcome. Skills for Care (2007: 4) define 'supervision' as 'an accountable process which supports, assures and develops the knowledge skills and values of an individual, group or team'. ODPs have not as a profession yet formalized their approach towards clinical supervision but it has advantages for registered professionals, who need to meet set standards such as the regulatory standards.

ODPs who are in advanced roles working outside of theatres and with wider multidisciplinary teams may already be familiar with clinical supervision. However this is still in the early stages of development within theatres. ODPs therefore need to develop clinical supervision to support each other, especially as the perioperative environment is a stressful environment to work in. To ensure clinical supervision is effective therefore, it is important that a safe and confidential process is developed within the perioperative environment to support and develop the ODP and their colleagues to discuss and express opinions on aspects of their work and how they can improve or develop these further. The benefits of developing this process of clinical supervision within the perioperative environment are threefold – to the practitioner, team and the patient.

* The individual ODP can benefit as it will enable them to reflect and challenge their own practice, gain feedback from peers and can contribute to their professional development. It complements the continual professional development requirements of the regulator and provides ODPs with new avenues of development that can be achieved by working with others.
* The whole team benefits by gaining a sense of value and therefore the chance to develop a shared culture to work within. This works best if there is an established benchmark of behaviours and openness to identify skill deficits within a team and how a greater understanding of each other's roles and responsibilities can improve the working practices of all. It also enables those who feel

they need or want more support to express this and discuss how this can be achieved and shared within the team in a non-judgemental, safe environment.

• Ultimately the patient who comes to theatre benefits the most as they will receive high-quality care as the ultimate aim of clinical supervision is the improvement of practice. The patient will also be cared for by staff who are supportive of each other and are able to manage the emotional, personal and professional aspects of their practice and thus are a more effective team.

The most effective approaches/models for clinical supervision are either one-to-one or group supervision. The one-to-one methods are more familiar within theatres particularly for the newly qualified practitioners. Successful supervision of the newly qualified practitioner will lead to a greater sense of self-confidence in their ability to understand and learn the responsibility of their role and help with the difficult challenges at this stage in their professional development and will assure them that there is a robust support structure. The key to successful clinical supervision however is not to get stuck using one method without exploring others to ensure that the process is effective.

When commencing clinical supervision, it should initially be made clear that it is all about support and development and not a covert way of performance managing someone. There are other tools available for this and it is about using the right approach to manage each situation. It is also important to set expectations and establish ground rules, most importantly relating to honesty and trust that must be maintained at all times. The focus is to create a safe environment to allow ODPs to reflect on and develop their practice without feeling it is always subject to scrutiny. The clinical supervision process relies on the good relationships between the supervisor and those they are supervising.

The supervisor should have appropriate qualifications, knowledge and skills in the area of practice where they will undertake their supervisory role. In addition they also need to have essential non-clinical skills such as good interpersonal skills, problem-solving skills and be able to give effective and timely feedback. The supervisor should also be a role model in maintaining their own professional development and also seek supervision of their practice and roles they are undertaking. The supervisor needs to be clear on the type/model of supervision they are embarking on with the individual or group. It is important that that they are supportive and approachable; aware of the individuals' or group's experience and skills, identify personal and professional development needs; keep records of the sessions and review any plans made and ensure they are actioned in the specified time. Both the supervisor and supervisee need to understand that any issues that arise regarding concerns on conduct, competence and health regarding an ODP will need to be shared and managed appropriately; and these may be managed outside the supervision process.

ODPs undertaking supervision (the supervisee) should be active rather than passive and hence should prepare for the sessions by identifying areas of their practice they wish to discuss. They should keep records of their sessions and take responsibility for completing the agreed actions, which could form part of what needs to be further discussed at development reviews/appraisals.

**Stop and think**

What areas of your practice would you like to openly discuss on a one to one or within a group that would benefit your personal and professional development and care provided to the patient?

## Recognizing and managing stress

The ODP will encounter stressful situations in the perioperative environment and therefore needs to develop an effective mechanism to identify and manage their stress. The stressful situations may manifest themselves from a number of triggers within the team; for example, relating to technical equipment, personal or patient problems, teamwork issues, distractions and difficulty with time management. It may also arise from other factors such as a death in the perioperative environment or the highly emotional aspect of caring for terminally ill children who come to theatre. A number of these are not within the control of the ODP and can have a significant impact on the performance of the individual and the team. While patient safety is paramount and technical skills are developed at a high-performance level, these are not the only factors that the ODP should consider as part of their role. It is worth noting at this point that it is often the non-technical skills of communication, situation awareness, leadership and poor decision-making skills that can lead to poor outcomes for patients.

The ODP must therefore be self-aware of their own stress as an important part of being a professional as the more stressed an individual becomes, the greater the risk will be of them making a mistake. It can be hard for the ODP to recognize stress as this can manifest itself in a variety of ways. Stress is not an illness but a state; however, if it continues for a long period it can develop into psychological, mental and physical symptoms. The causes of stress can be due to the demand of the workload and lack of control to express this. It could be the lack of support or changes to your role or the environment and those you work with. But equally the stress could come from personal problems, finance, bereavement, divorce, childcare, moving house and a wide variety of health issues either personally or relationship related.

Stress should not always be viewed as negative within the operating theatre as the ODP may find that an individual stressful situation; for example, an emergency case enables them to work particularly effectively. However, debriefing from these stressful cases is important both as a valuable learning event and an ability to help both the team and individual manage these stressful times better in the future. The impact of day-to-day-stress, such as workload, needs to be managed by the ODP to ensure that it does not adversely affect their wellbeing. The ODP needs to be able to recognize the emotional symptoms of stress as these can create negative or depressive feelings that may leave the ODP doubting whether they can cope and questioning their abilities. This can lead to a loss of motivation, commitment and confidence that can manifest itself in mood swings with an increase of emotional reactions like being more tearful, sensitive, aggressive and feelings of loneliness and becoming withdrawn. This can cause mental dysfunction that can present as poor memory, confusion, indecision and the inability to concentrate. Stress can also see changes in behaviour such as eating habits and sleeping patterns or an increase in alcohol consumption or smoking as this is often used as a way of coping. It is essential that the ODP can recognize and identify their stress and assess the impact upon their practice and health, as ODPs have a professional responsibility to ensure their fitness to practise.

The ODP therefore needs to be aware of these signs of stress and also know what to do about it especially if their stress is exacerbated by their work. Patient Safety First produced a useful document in 2010, *Implementing Human Factors in Healthcare*, which discusses stress and coping mechanisms and this is a useful resource for ODPs. Initially, the ODP should speak with their line manager, trade union or human resources at the earliest possible sign of stress to see what support is available to alleviate, reduce or stop the symptoms. It should be recognized that many of these symptoms may also be an indication of other health issues and therefore seeking advice from your doctor is important.

In the operating theatre it is hard to prevent stress but there are many things the ODP can do to manage it more effectively, such as taking exercise, reviewing their time management, speaking to their line manager to gain their support; for example, maybe by some changes in work pattern. This could be a simple request to ensure they have a lunch break that allows them to leave the department for lunch thus helping the individual with gaining control of their workload by compartmentalizing it so it is divided into manageable sessions. If there are external issues, taking some annual leave to concentrate on the matter in hand maybe helpful as may the advice available though many agencies or the General Practitioner (GP). Recognizing the early signs of stress will help prevent it getting worse and from leading to further health problems. The ODP's health is paramount in dealing with patients and therefore management of stress is a crucial aspect of professional responsibility and it is the ODP's responsibility to ensure that they discuss matters early with their line manager or personal tutor.

### Stop and think

Think about an occasion when you experienced a period of tension/stress. This may have been when you had a number of deadlines to meet or a number of personal issues in addition to your work; or maybe a very high pressure event. Think about how you knew you were stressed, how did those signs of stress manifest themselves? Now think about what you did or could have done to rectify this.

## Communication within the team

This section will not be dealing with the fundamental theories of communication, as there are many texts that approach this and they are often threaded and themed through academic courses. It is a key skill that the ODP needs to be taught and assessed upon, understand, develop and reflect upon to see how best to promote better communication during their professional life. It is important to realize that not everyone shares the same preferred communication style. Allen and Brock (2000) cites the Myers–Briggs Type Indicator (MBTI) as being widely used in education and training to understand personality types, and although everyone is unique there are certain behavioural traits that are common, predictable and consistent.

Communication skills are a vital part of the role of the ODP and should take a learned approach, which is simple but clear, as it underpins good care. It is the foundation of dealing with colleagues, patients and their carers. Effective communication relies on all our skills not only to build trust but also to work well with others benefiting from the patient accessing healthcare. In 2000 Greco et al. identified 10 attributes that patients look for in healthcare professionals:

- being greeted warmly;
- listened to;
- clear explanations;
- reassurance;
- confidence in the ability of the staff;
- able to express their concerns and fears;
- respected;
- given time;
- consideration given to personal circumstances when seeking advice or treatment;
- being treated like a person not just a disease.

These aspects are still current in today's health delivery as seen in many reports where patients have raised concerns.

The ODP has a significant role in managing the message to the patient and others within the perioperative team. In the perioperative environment there are many factors that affect the flow of information such as interruptions, team familiarity, unpredictable incidents and changes to schedules. It has been cited in many cases where errors have occurred where the root cause has been communication failures and errors. In order to improve communications the development of briefings and timeout have become a part of the perioperative preparation routine.

There are three related levels that affect the team in the operating theatres regarding communication:

- the nature of the task that needs to be done;
- the procedure to ensure the task is performed effectively;
- the interpersonal relationship of those in the team.

There are a number of unavoidable barriers that affect communication within the perioperative environment; one being wearing hats and surgical masks, which can create difficulty in hearing or distortion of the message or even misinterpretation for example because the 'listener' is unable to see the lip movement. Familiar terminology can also be a barrier; it is frequently used by those who work within the perioperative team, such as various names for different types of swabs, abbreviations and acronyms, which is like a unique code that alienates others who are not familiar. Cultural variation in language can also contribute to being a barrier in the message being received and transmitted and the ODP should be aware of the impact of cultural considerations in communication. The ODP will recognize how the team dynamics play an important role in setting the scene for the surgical procedure and the care to be delivered. The theatre environment is generally quiet but there are contributing noises that can interfere with how a message is transmitted and received; for example, if the surgeon, or the awake patient wishes to have music playing; technological noises like ventilators; monitors, suction and surgical equipment such as power tools can all impact on the distortion of effective communication.

It is equally important to communicate an effective message when providing written records of care for the patient when receiving and transferring of their care within the perioperative environment. All these forms should be clear and legible using no jargon and ensuring those in receipt of the information understand it appropriately. Abbreviations are to be avoided unless they are recognized terminology used by all. This is crucial, particularly when the patient is being moved from one care setting to another. The quality in the continuity of care provided by the many teams that the patient will experience relies heavily on the interpersonal skills and the effective sharing of appropriate information both verbally and through the written records of care.

The patient's view of their care will be affected by the interpersonal skills and the interaction they have with the ODP. Therefore the non-verbal communication gestures used can be discouraging for the patient especially where they are greeted by someone who, for example, during the anaesthetic phase leans against the workstation with folded arms thus giving the message of not being bothered with them. Likewise, the team dashing about can relay the message that it is very busy, maybe too busy and, the patient may neglect to ask questions or share important information feeling that they do not want to 'be a burden' to an already busy team. The team need to recognize these approaches and raise them in the appropriate forum so that they are more patient sensitive in the perioperative environment. Teams need to look at their approaches to communication and the potential impact this can have on not only the patient but different levels of staff who can be equally affected.

**Stop and think**

Have you ever noticed how communication has increased or distracted from the progression of the operation. Think about a situation where maybe there has been a stressful moment, either before or during the operation, where an interruption, bleeding or lack of or malfunction of equipment has occurred. Reflect on what aspect of communication could have improved the outcome?

### Active listening

The term 'active listening' is often used by many healthcare professionals to stress the importance of the need to listen, and not merely to the words being spoken but also to the many complex layers the person speaking is relaying to you. The listening skill will vary depending on the context and the matter in hand. In the operating theatre the ODP may need to elicit important information that is crucial to the task in hand, whether this is taking down vital signs to be reported to another or gathering patient specific information for use in their care. The use of good questioning technique can be supportive to active listening, such as the use of open or closed question, which will encourage a certain response depending on the information needed. By using these it can support other tools in effective communication.

### Using the SBAR tool to aid communication in the perioperative team

The perioperative environment is dynamic in nature and this results in a number of potential risks especially if essential information is not adequately communicated. It is therefore essential that ODPs are able to convey pertinent information effectively. To support all healthcare practitioners, including ODPs, in communicating information the SBAR tool has been developed to ensure that the practitioner has a structure for conveying the key points relating to a patient's care. SBAR is an acronym of Situation, Background, Assessment and Recommendation and a worked example will demonstrate how this is used.

The nature of the clinical environment and interventions means that ODPs are caring for patients who may exhibit a rapid change in their physiological state, both during and after surgery; consequently ODPs need to be able to identify that there is cause for concern and raise this effectively in a timely manner. It is therefore essential that all relevant information is handed over to other practitioners within the team and especially if there are any concerns that these are communicated effectively. To aid ODPs in doing this the National Health Service (NHS) Institute for Innovation and Improvement (2008) advocate the use of the SBAR tool to ensure that essential information is shared in a clear and concise manner and this can be used to inform verbal or written communications at any point in the patent journey. The steps in using SBAR for communications are as follows and will be illustrated using an example of an ODP raising a concern with a medic regarding a patent in the post-anaesthetic care unit (PACU).

The ODP should initially describe the *situation*. This includes identifying yourself, that is particularly important in the perioperative environment when all staff wear the same attire and even though you may 'know' another colleague on a conversational basis, they may not be aware of your professional background. The situation also includes an explanation of the patient and the cause for concern. For example: 'This is ODP Alexa Berry from the post-anaesthetic care unit in main theatres. I am calling about Mrs Kelly from the gynaecology list this afternoon, she has been in PACU for 1 hour and has become increasingly tachycardic, she is also tachypneic and hypotensive.' This concise summary immediately informs the other person of whom they are speaking to and the reason for the call and has therefore 'set the scene' for the conversation.

The second stage is the *background* that will help the medic gain a full picture of the patient, especially as you may be talking to a member of the on-call surgical team rather that the team who actually operated on the patient. When you explain the patient's background you need to include why the patient was admitted, relevant medical history and the medical background. This is important so that the listener can start to consider the situation and again allows the conversation to be more effective. In an environment where there are a number of time pressures, practitioners should try to make each conversation effective; for example there would be no value in describing a case and a medic issuing a verbal prescription to then be told the patient is allergic to that drug and so including all this information at this stage allows the listener to start to build a complete 'picture' of the patient.

For example: 'Mrs Kelly is a 45-year-old woman who was admitted this morning for an elective vaginal hysterectomy. She had a spinal anaesthetic and it is noted that she was a potentially difficult intubation. All her pre-operative investigations were normal and she has no allergies. She was on hormone replacement therapy that she stopped 4 weeks before surgery.' In this example the ODP has provided a summary of all the relevant medical history; the medic now knows that Mrs Kelly was otherwise fit and well and that should she need to return to theatre she has the potential to be difficult to intubate.

The next stage requires the ODP to report their *assessment* of the case; this will include vital signs and clinical assessment. The ODP should have assimilated their clinical assessment with other objective measures and considered the potential cause for concern, thus demonstrating the need for ODPs to have good skills of patient assessment and a comprehensive understanding of anatomy and physiology. For example: 'Mrs Kelly is tachycardic with a weak, thready pulse of 110 beats per minute, her blood pressure is 75/50 mmHG, her respiration rate is 28, she has not produced any urine in the last hour and she is cool and clammy to the touch. She is exhibiting signs of hypovolaemic shock and I think she might be bleeding internally.' This assessment has clearly indicated the severity of Mrs Kelly's condition and the ODP has offered a suggestion of what they believe the cause may be based on their clinical assessment.

The final stage requires the ODP to make a *recommendation*. This is not a recommendation specifically for clinical care but rather it is what you need to achieve by the end of the conversation. This may be instructions for what actions the ODP needs to take; for example, this may be preparing equipment or receiving a verbal prescription. In order to make this recommendation, the ODP needs to be clear about what they require from the other person and should end the conversation with clearly agreed actions. For example: 'I think you need to come and see Mrs Kelly. How soon can you get here? Would you like me to order blood products/arrange for the emergency theatre to be on standby?' In this way the ODP has said what they require (the medic to review Mrs Kelly) and has an indication of when the medic will be arriving and what they can do in the interim period to prepare for the subsequent care of the patient, based on the presentation and initial assessment.

SBAR has been shown to be a structured way to share information with other team members and these four elements are important for any handover. The example has shown SBAR in a telephone conversation to raise a concern about a deteriorating patient and shows how the essential information can be communicated succinctly to brief another professional on a patient's clinical condition. The four elements of SBAR however can be equally well applied to other handover situations as it ensures that all of the key patient information has been communicated and therefore ODPs should ensure that they are familiar with this tool.

### Stop and think

Could you use this SBAR to ensure you communicate all relevant information in other handovers? For example at shift change – you may want to think about using the recommendations to explain what is still needed. Try to write an SBAR in the anaesthetic role when handing over a patient undergoing a complex procedure to the next shift.

## Conclusion

This chapter has explored the many facets of the perioperative team and the complexity of working in a team that is dynamic and hence constantly evolving and developing. This constant development requires the ODP to be an adaptive team member able to modify their behaviour to integrate within the team, while retaining their professional identify and asserting their professional knowledge. In order to achieve this effectively the ODP needs a good level of self-awareness to be able to recognize both their input to the team and that of others. The focus of the perioperative team will always be the delivery of high-quality care to the patient and therefore the team needs to ensure that the specific goals to achieve this are articulated and agreed. This is essential to enable the team as a whole, and hence the ODP, to work effectively as a team towards a shared goal.

## Key points

- To work effectively teams must have a clear goal that has been agreed by the team.
- Effective communication is a vital component of professional responsibility and the ODP needs to be able to recognize the barriers to this and address them appropriately.
- Professional wellbeing is paramount to being a competent practitioner caring for those in their care.
- Clinical supervision can provide support to and develop the ODP as part of their ongoing professional development.

## References and further reading

Allen, J. and Brock, S.A. (2000) *Healthcare Communication Using Personality Type*. London: Routledge.

Borill, C., West, M., Rees, A., Dawson, J., Shapiro, D., Richards, A., Carletta, J. and Garrard, S. (2001) *The Effectiveness of Health Care Teams in the National Health Service*. Available online at http://homepages.inf.ed.ac.uk/jeanc/DOH-final-report.pdf (accessed 25 November 2013).

Greco, M., Brownlea, A., McGovern, J. and Cavanagh, M. (2000) 'Consumers as educators: implementation of patient feedback in general practice training', *Health Communications*, 12 (1): 73–93.

Health Care Development Agency (2003) *Teamworking Guide for Primary Healthcare*. Available online at http://www.nice.org.uk/aboutnice/whoweare/aboutthehda/hdapublications/hda_publications.jsp?o=225 (accessed 25 November 2013).

Health Care Professions Council (HCPC) (2014) *Standards of Proficiency for Operating Department Practitioners*. London: HCPC.

National Health Service (NHS) Institute for Innovation and Improvement (2008) *SBAR – Situation-Background-Assessment-Recommendation*. Available online at http://www.institute.nhs.uk/quality_and_service_improvement_tools/quality_and_service_improvement_tools/sbar_-_situation_-_background_-_assessment_-_recommendation.html (accessed 3 November 2013).

Patient Safety First (2010) *Implementing Human Factors in Healthcare – How to Guide*. Available online at www.patientsafetyfirst.nhs.uk (accessed 30 November 2013).

Skills for Care (2007) *Providing Effective Supervision: A Workforce Development Tool, Including a Unit of Competence and Supporting Guidance*. Available online at http://www.skillsforcare.org.uk/publications/ProvidingEffectiveSupervision.aspx (accessed 2 November 2013).

Tuckman, B. (1965) 'Developmental sequence in small groups', *Psychological Bulletin*, 63 (6): 384–99.

# 2 Developing your learning as an Operating Department Practitioner

## Andrew Gulley

*Andrew Gulley*

---

**Key topics**

- Exploring learning styles and theories
- How to use learning outcomes to enhance your learning

- Assessment and revision strategies
- Tools to support learning including portfolios

---

## Introduction

The aim of this chapter is to take you through a back to basics perspective on teaching, learning and assessment approaches used in higher education (HE) for both new learners and those practitioners returning to learning. The skills, practices and attitudes fundamental to operating department practice are learned from the achievement, integration and critical application of knowledge and understanding, cognitive/intellectual skills, key/transferable skills and practical skills gained from the whole of the educational experience (College of Operating Department Practitioners (CODP), 2011).

By linking the learning styles, theories and assessment explored in this chapter, you will be able to develop effective learning plans, strategies and behaviours to meet professional standards and ultimately be successful in your studies. It is acknowledged that some content will already be known to the experienced learner; however, the focus of the chapter is to support all Operating Department Practitioner (ODP) learners in their ongoing professional education.

## Why is this relevant?

Whether you are new or returning to learning there needs to be some adjustments to how you plan your time, or to the new experience of life at university, which can be can be complex and confusing. There will be many challenges, barriers and difficulties you will have to face in order to be a successful learner. Studying operating department practice brings with it a unique set of other challenges; for example, the whole learning experience of clinical practice, sometimes viewed as the vocational aspect of the curriculum where the learner links academic theory and knowledge to their application in practice. When undertaking your ODP pre- or post-registration studies you will have to fit academic study around clinical placement hours, or clinical shift patterns.

With this limited amount of time for studying, it is important that any learner understands the approaches to teaching, learning and assessment so that they are not perceived as barriers to success due to ambiguity and misapprehension, but moreover are understood and engaged with effectively to enhance the development of their own learning and personal development; hence learning to learn. By understanding these approaches, the skills, practices and attitudes fundamental to operating department practice, then the whole of the educational experience will become pleasant and engaging, and not develop into a period of 'study with tears', but with 'cheers'. This chapter provides learners with an insight and understanding of the key academic norms and values relating to teaching, learning and assessment primarily in the HE setting; however, these skills of learning are central to your ongoing development throughout your career as an ODP.

## Learning styles

ODPs will all assimilate and process information in different ways and within a diverse group of learners, there will equally be a diverse range of learning 'styles'. Many people recognize that each learner, and to some degree the learner themselves, prefers different learning styles and teaching techniques in order to be able grasp the subject in both academic and clinical practice settings (D'Amore et al., 2011). While studying you may learn material in a number of different ways; for example, by seeing and hearing, reflecting and acting on your learning, thinking logically and instinctively, and analysing and visualizing the information being presented. This should be in a continuous manner to ensure that development takes place in a progressive way measured against your learning objectives. These regular successes are important as they allow recognition of achievement and build confidence in your abilities to succeed.

Learning styles group common characteristics in learning that help you learn effectively. They also change the way in which we internally represent experiences, the way we recall information, and even the words we choose, all of which has a bearing on assessment outcomes and achievements. Having an insight into learning styles can help you develop appropriate strategies to improve individual academic development and performance (Horton et al., 2012).

## The VARK learning styles model

Acquisition of knowledge through experience is associated with different learning styles, and here we consider the concepts of visual, auditory, reading/writing and kinaesthetic modes of learning (VARK) (Fleming, 2012) and those of Kolb (1984). Fleming (2012) suggests that the VARK modalities appear to reflect the lifelong learning experiences of learners. The VARK leaning styles inventory not only tells you what your preferred style is, but also offers specific strategies for teaching, learning, revision and assessment. In a classroom setting or in the operating theatre, you will be using your senses to assimilate and process information in different ways. In the classroom setting, for example, the tutor may present an image of an anatomical structure or they may talk about a patient care situation. In contrast, in the perioperative environment, you might look at and identify specific internal anatomy. Whichever context or situation of the learning experience, you will be using some form of sensory modality; that is: Visual (seeing the image), Aural (listening to your mentor/tutor), Read/write (taking notes in a lecture) and Kinaesthetic activity (hands-on care).

The VARK modalities, characteristics and examples of learning strategies are shown in Table 2.1. Kolb's (1984) model draws on the cognitive personality styles assessed for example by the classic Myers–Briggs type indicator, a psychological personality test that has been used for over 50 years

**Stop and think**

Look at the VARK table and consider which of these techniques you have used for learning in the past? Or if you have not studied for a while, how do you best remember things? Consider how you can use this important information about your own learning to support your studies.

**Table 2.1** The VARK modalities and characteristics

| Mode | Characteristics |
| --- | --- |
| Visual | This preference includes the depiction of information in maps, spider diagrams, charts, graphs, flow charts, labelled diagrams, symbolic arrows, circles, prefers symbols to represent words |
| Auditory | This is a preference for information that is heard or spoken. Learns best from lectures, group discussion, radio, email, using mobile phones, speaking, web-chat and talking things through |
| Reading/ writing | This preference emphasizes text-based input and output – reading and writing in all its forms, but especially manuals, reports, essays and assignments |
| Kinaesthetic | A preference related to the use of experience and practice (simulated or real). A strong preference to learn from the experience of doing something |

*Source:* adapted from Fleming (2012).

and has gone through extensive validity and reliability studies (D'Amore et al., 2011) (see Table 2.2). As an ODP you will probably engage with all of Kolb's learning styles; for example, using simulation in Advanced Trauma Life Support (Activist) or linking your lecture notes to practice (Theorist).

Throughout a programme of study there will generally be a balance of teaching and learning methods and therefore all learners will have an opportunity to learn in their preferred learning style. The balance will also mean the learner will be exposed to an approach, which they may not prefer, but provides a set of new learning strategies, which they may not initially be comfortable with, but may be beneficial in being successful in their academic and vocational studies. Individual learners have preferred learning styles that influence and guide their learning. If you have an insight into your learning style you can develop appropriate strategies to improve your academic development. The VARK and Kolb models, although not exclusively, provide a comprehensive analysis of a learner's learning style and suggested learning strategies, but should only be used as an aid and not a prescriptive method of learning. In the author's experience, this model has a proven track record for academic success (Richardson, 2011).

**Table 2.2** Kolb's learning styles and characteristics

| Learning style | Characteristics and preferred study/learning activities |
| --- | --- |
| Activist | Active experimentation via simulations, case study, homework |
| Reflector | Reflective observations through logs, journals, thought cascading |
| Theorist | Abstract conceptualization; for example, lectures |
| Pragmatist | Concrete experience such as observations, application to practice |

*Source:* adapted from D'Amore et al. (2011).

**Stop and think**

Thinking back to your own experiences, what type of learning sessions have you found most beneficial?

Look at Kolb's learning styles and characteristics and identify how your own preferences relate to the different styles that Kolb suggests.

## Kolb's model of experiential learning

As an ODP a lot of your learning will be drawn from you educational and practice experiences. You can further develop the learning gained from these experiences if you identify where you are in terms of your learning cycle. Kolb's (1984) model of experiential learning presents learning as a process whereby knowledge is created through the transformations of experiences in a cycle. This model fits well with the profession's body of knowledge, identified in the pre-registration ODP curriculum, which advocates that cognitive/intellectual skills, key/transferable skills and practical skills are gained from the whole of the educational experience (CODP, 2011).

Kolb's theory provides a rationale for a variety of learning methods including: independent learning; learning by doing; work-based learning; and problem-based learning. These methods are all necessary if learning is to be consolidated and implemented in practice. As you move through the cycle you first have the immediate experience that leads to observations and reflections on the experience. These reflections are then assimilated and linked with previous knowledge and translated into abstract concepts or theories, which result in new ways and actions to adjust to the experience that can be tested and explored. Kolb describes the cycle of experiential learning as four stages (see Figure 2.1).

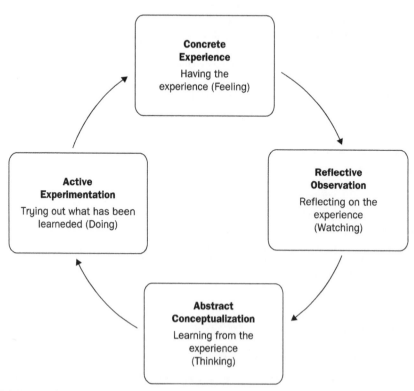

**Figure 2.1** Kolb's learning cycle.
*Source:* adapted from Kolb (1984)

By using the Kolb's cycle as an example consider an ODP who has cared for a very anxious patient undergoing general anaesthesia (concrete experience). After dealing with this anxious patient, the ODP reflects upon what took place (reflective observation), and discusses this with their mentor/ other colleagues. The ODP then considers this in the context of their previous experiences and published policies, good practice and literature (abstract conceptualization). Based upon these reflections and wider reading the ODP then identifies some strategies of change that they can apply to similar clinical situations in the future (active experimentation). They can then assess the efficacy of these strategies by working through the cycle again.

## Educational learning theories

The use of educational learning theories can inform teaching strategies and the selection of different learning resources. Ultimately, the learning activities in which the learner actually engages will determine what they will actually learn.

There are four common educational theories that can be clearly applied to operating department practice education.

### Behaviourist theory

Behaviourist theory is primarily and historically associated with Pavlov's dogs ('classical conditioning') and Skinner's rats ('operant conditioning') (Sarafino, 2008). Most of the experiments and evidence for this theory are derived from animals and then generalized to human behaviours, and therefore it is open to criticism. Pavlov and Skinner worked on the idea that if you repeated the same stimulus enough times and gave a negative reinforcement (electric shock) or positive reinforcement (food) for incorrect and correct action, eventually your subject would 'learn'. In an educational setting, behaviour theory or behaviourism implies that the tutor/mentor provides the negative or positive reinforcement of the behaviour to the learner. Reinforcement or punishment and reward continue in behaviour theory, although it is more politically correct to call them feedback, and to use positive rather than negative methods (Hutchinson, 2007). In ODP education, the behaviour theory is relevant mainly to the development of clinical skills through simulation.

Clinical skills can be taught by breaking them down into steps, and each step and the whole sequence are rehearsed in a safe environment. Feedback is given to modify the behaviour; for example, a learner scrubs up for the first time, but their scrubs are soaking wet. The mentor can then modify the behaviour by demonstrating or suggesting another method of scrubbing that would keep them dry. The learner then adopts this behaviour as a result of the feedback (reinforcement) and reflection on their performance and successfully scrubs without getting wet (learning). Clearly this can be seen in Kolb's cycle of experiential learning.

### Cognitive theory

The theorists of the twentieth century believed that we learn by receiving information, processing it, storing it and then later retrieving it for use. Processing the information means you repeat it, use it, apply it, and try a number of formats. Learning comes from understanding therefore organization and structure of teaching contributes to learning. The discovery of knowledge or constructing meaning is central to learning.

We can see cognitive theory in practice in a classroom setting. You are given information, perhaps some individual problem solving or group work that you work through with applied examples. The teaching is planned, organized and takes into account individual perceptions and differences (learning styles). You process the information, store it and later retrieve the information for use in an exam or discussion in practice.

Cognitive feedback is an integral part of cognitive theory, similar to the reinforcement of behaviourism. For example, your mentor will provide you with constructive and organized feedback on your performance in practice. You will hopefully understand and identify your strengths and weakness and adapt your practice accordingly.

From cognitive theory we can also examine the concepts of surface and deep leaning approaches.

## Surface learning

This is the storing of lots of information in the short-term memory for a specific purpose; for example, a written examination. It leads to superficial retention of material (unprocessed) for examinations and does not promote understanding or long-term retention of knowledge and information; for example, cramming for an exam. To be able to understand and apply your learning, a deep learning approach is required.

## Deep learning

This process involves the critical analysis of new ideas, linking them to already known concepts and principles, and leads to understanding and long-term retention of concepts so that they can be used for problem solving in unfamiliar situations (Higher Education Authority (HEA), 2011). It assumes learning will be banked in long-term memory store as it has been learned, examined, considered, applied and understood. Table 2.3 summarizes the differences between surface and deep approaches to learning.

---

**Stop and think**

By looking at Table 2.3 can you identify which one represents your current approach to learning?

Think about the different elements of ODP professional knowledge – do you see, for example, anatomy and physiology as separate to your anaesthetic, surgical and post-anaesthetic care knowledge?

Or do you link all these aspects together in order to analyse the patient care?

---

**Table 2.3** The characteristics in surface and deep approaches to learning

| Surface learning characteristics | Deep learning characteristics |
| --- | --- |
| • Relying on rote learning | • Looking for meaning |
| • Focusing on outwards signs and the formulae needed to solve a problem | • Focusing on the central argument or concepts needed to solve a problem. |
| • Receiving information passively | • Interacting actively |
| • Failing to distinguish principles from examples | • Distinguishing between argument and evidence |
| • Treating parts of modules and programmes as separate | • Making connections between different modules |
| • Not recognizing new material as building on previous work | • Relating new and previous knowledge |
| • Seeing course content simply as material to be learned for the exam | • Linking course content to practice |

*Source:* adapted from HEA (2011)

### Strategic learning

Strategic learning is recognized as an approach where the learner strategically streamlines their study to obtain higher grades and hence is usually assessment driven. This approach however is not beneficial to your development as a professional as it may result in the omission of key information that could be to the detriment of your clinical knowledge.

### Humanist theory

Humanist learning is student centred and personalized, with the aim of developing self-actualized people in a co-operative, supportive environment. This theory suggests that learning is a natural process and comes from within. Motivation, purpose and learning objectives are important aspects that promote effective learning. However, you need to consider that you are an individual human being and that a social situation may affect your learning; for example, a domestic situation may impact your learning. Furthermore, anxiety and emotion affect learning and your behaviour; for example, if you lack confidence working alongside a particular consultant surgeon, this may be exacerbated by your personal stress. However, the positive aspects of the humanist theory are relevance and motivation. For example, being given responsibility aids learning, a mentor may say 'you run today's operating list', which allows you to develop you own skills and confidence.

## Learning outcomes

Learning outcomes specify the intended endpoint of a period of study activities. They should ideally clearly indicate the nature or level of learning required to achieve them successfully. They should be achievable in a given time and assessed by an appropriate method. The language used should be clear to learners; this will relate to explicit statements of achievement and will always contain verbs, words that will express actions, events or expected behaviours (Quality Assurance Agency (QAA), 2007).

The use of learning outcomes is an integral part of the academic infrastructure, deriving from curriculum competencies, subject benchmark statements and the framework for HE qualifications; these are integrated in programme and module specifications (QAA, 2012; CODP, 2009). Learning outcomes, both academic and clinical, are intended to enhance learning across a wide range of skills, which include the development of knowledge and understanding, cognitive/intellectual skills, key transferable and practical skills. They provide information about the content to be learned and the way in which you will have to demonstrate satisfactory knowledge and enabling you to make more appropriate choices about study methods and relevant content. Learning outcomes also facilitate evaluation of your learning as they are integral to the assessment process and criteria for assessment. For example, you can write and agree specific personal learning objectives with your mentors to target weaker area of practice. As a registered ODP you can use learning outcomes to address your personal development plans and continual professional development needs.

For example, individual learning outcomes relate to one of the three domains described by Bloom's taxonomy (Mobbs, 2012) depending on the nature of what level of cognition (understanding) is being assessed. These are:

- the cognitive domain (knowledge and intellectual skills);
- the psychomotor domain (physical skills, clinical practice);
- the domain of professional behaviours (feelings and attitudes) (Cassidy, 2009).

During the course of learning, learners will develop and attain different levels of cognitive, psychomotor and professional skills. Bloom classically identified six levels within the cognitive domain, from the simple recall or recognition of facts, as the lowest level, through increasingly more complex and abstract mental levels, to the highest order that is classified as evaluation (Bloom, 1994). These levels can also be applied to the psychomotor and professional behaviour domains. Bloom's taxonomy of the hierarchy of cognitive domains, descriptions and the associated verbs are often used in learning outcomes. Each domain has associated verbs or statements that are integrated into learning outcomes at different stages with an educational programme.

By setting clearly articulated learning outcomes/objectives, the ODP can develop metacognitive skills (knowing about knowing). These skills aid you in reflecting upon and self-directing your thinking and learning processes. You can use course learning outcomes and clinical practice outcomes to monitor and evaluate your academic and clinical practice skills and progression. Ultimately, manage and develop your own learning more effectively.

## Revision strategies

Revising for an exam is one of the most individualized processes within academic life. There are many texts on the subject of how to revise and prepare for examinations. This chapter therefore provides an applied insight into some useful guidance for ODP students.

The unique nature of ODP education means that these students are often undertaking clinical practice while preparing for exams that can lead to stress for some learners. A little stress however can be positive and can contribute to good psychological preparation. When experiencing too much physical or mental stress the body increases its adrenaline levels, which gives rise to feelings of anxiety and tension and can have a negative impact on revision and exam performance (humanist learning theory again). Being fully prepared is generally considered the most effective way to overcome stress and anxiety about exams.

There are three revision strategies that have been shown to be useful to learners who have found traditional methods ineffective: being organized; using mind maps; reducing notes and using mobile technology.

### Being organized

Burns and Sinfield (2012) suggest that having revision action plans adds discipline to your studies and ensures that you exploit and get control of your revision thereby reducing stress. You should consider how the suggested actions in Table 2.4 can potentially help you in organizing your revision and preparing for exams.

**Table 2.4** An action plan for revision

| Activity | Examples |
| --- | --- |
| Positive state of mind | Being motivated, positive messages, healthy lifestyle, accepting the challenge |
| Time | Engaging with revision early, organizing study time effectively, optimizing time, setting priorities |
| Variety | Study in short spells, use various techniques, make things interesting |
| Over-learning | Rewrite notes, make flash cards, essay, plans, creative trigger. |
| Practice | Do past questions, engage with extended materials and set mock exam conditions |
| People | Share revision with others, study buddies |
| Selection | What topics do I need to be revising? What level of detail do I need in the exam? |

*Source:* adapted from Burns and Sinfield (2012)

## Using mind maps

A mind map, or thought mapping, encourages the left and right hemispheres of the brain to integrate more; subsequently, this improves memory. The left side of the brain is where the logical thinking occurs whereas the right side has a more creative style; however, the brain uses both hemispheres to memorize information. The constructs of a mind map are ideally suited to encourage both halves of the brain to work better together and make learning easier.

A mind map is a powerful non-linear (written sentences and phrases going left to right down a page) graphic technique that harnesses the full range of cortical skills such as words, images, number, logic, rhythm, colour and spatial awareness. This is achieved in a single, uniquely influential manner and can give you an overview of a large subject or topic area. Mind maps can collect and hold large amounts of data and illustrate the links between different aspects of the topic. They also encourage active planning techniques by allowing you to see links and make connections. It is visually stimulating and aids concentration and memory. Mind maps can be applied to any topic that you are studying; these include planning essays, reports and presentations, revision and note-taking tasks.

You can create your own maps quickly and effectively on a piece of A4 notepaper using coloured pens, but if you prefer there are a number of software programs freely available in universities and the public domain that can create them for you. The use of colour, diagrams and images in mind mapping associates smaller bites of information and also encourages left- and right-side brain integration.

## The value of creating a précis

Learners can often be under the illusion that every handout, textbook article or web resource that is used on a course is as equally as important and therefore must be read and integrated. Creating a précis, a synopsis or summary of your notes and materials into more manageable resources will make learning less stressful. Organizing information into a series of memory triggers, and then reducing the number of triggers to a key word or image is a useful strategy. This can be seen in the mind map; for example, central topic, branch and sub-branches. Generally, learn the big things and summarize the smaller. The larger parts will act as rallying points to call the detailed abstract concepts to mind.

The rallying points are the triggers; they need not be images, but a 'mnemonic' for example. Mnemonic is another word for memory tool. Mnemonics are techniques for remembering information that is otherwise quite difficult to recall. They are a series of letters (an acronym) or words (usually a rhyme) used as triggers for recall of information, process, sequences, and so on. We probably remember the mnemonic for the colours of the rainbow. If you have just recalled it, isn't that a good indicator of how useful they are? The notes on the treble clef used in music is another common example; that is, 'FACE', the notes in between the lines and 'Every Good Boy Deserves Favour', the notes that fall on the lines. There are many medical mnemonics that learners can use to aid their recall of detailed information; for example, 'To Zanzibar By Motor Car' can be used for the five branches of the facial nerve – Temporal, Zygomatic, Buccal, Mandibular and Cervical.

### Stop and think

Mnemonics allow complex information to be condensed into a few words and essentially make your memory more efficient. They are no substitute for hard work and wider reading, but this is of little use if you cannot locate your facts or you get the information muddled up. Mnemonics allow you to secure information in your head with the aid of word play or visual associations.

Try creating mnemonics for:

- six functions of blood (factual exam revision);
- remembering the process for checking anaesthetic equipment (developing practice);
- the hierarchy of human needs (psychological theory).

## Using mobile technology to aid learning

The use of information technology has quickly become part of everyday life for most people in the developed world and is increasingly becoming an integral part of university life and the learning process. Trends in mobile technologies suggest that they have the potential to impact positively on learning in general and HE in particular (Nikoi, 2008). As technology advances, there will be associated advances in the usability of mobile devices for teaching, learning and assessment. If you conduct a search of a device's available applications for download, the results will demonstrate the increasing availability of educational material for learners. Potentially, learning may migrate to outside a classroom and lecture theatres into the learner's immediate environment (home or clinical placement) through the use of mobile devices.

A number of educators already use micro-blogs to create a community around a class or an activity. Educators who have used Twitter, for example, report that it is a useful feedback channel during and after class. After a lecture or seminar, tutors can encourage micro-blogging to support relationships among the people from the class and to further their learning. Teachers post tips of the day, questions, on writing assignments, and other prompts to keep learning going. Another popular use of Twitter and other micro-blogging sites is the building of professional networks. You can get to know other learning professionals, receive regular updates about professional practice, get help from experts, and even attract followers of your own.

Here are some practical thoughts on how to make the most of mobile devices, mp3 players, cameras, memory sticks or tablet devices when studying:

- Set up reminders for tutorials or assignments on the calendar.
- Create notes when you think of an idea for an assignment, or a question to ask your tutor.
- Photo or video a whiteboard diagram instead of copying it down.
- Record audio notes to summarize key points.
- Check your facts on the web: try the library resources for your subject area including websites, online journals and online books.
- Get help from others by phone or text.
- Access a dictionary or thesaurus online.
- Download audio or video files to your mp3 player.
- Use the calculator function.
- Subscribe to podcasts and radio programmes related to your course subject.
- Search the web for quizzes about your subject to check your understanding.
- Subscribe to Rich Site Summary (RSS) feeds of relevant information.

(adapted from the Open University, 2011)

### Recording lectures

Where a learner believes that there are good academic reasons to request permission to record a lecture to support their learning, there will be a local policy with which to comply with. The recording of classes or clinical practice and particularly sessions where patients and other learners are involved is generally not permitted. To fully realize the benefits and comply with the law, the HE institution must consider the rights of all relevant parties including students, staff, patients and carers, whose works, participation and content may appear within an audio or video recording (Joint Information Systems Committee (JISC), 2010). Copyright and data protection law under the Data Protection Act, 1998 (The National Archives, 2013) will be applicable where lectures, films, scripts, photographs, blogs and diagrams, for example, are being recorded. A recording is also a copyright work in its own right. You should also be aware that professional and regulatory standards apply to all your conduct at university and should be adhered to at all times and especially in the context of recording lectures.

### Professional aspects of mobile technology

Learners must courteously respect the use of personal mobile devices in relation to their use in the classroom or clinical placement setting. Furthermore, the growth and popularity of social networking websites makes it important for registered staff and learners to know how to use them without undermining their professional status. Ly (2010) reported that it appears to be quite easy to blur the line between an individual's professional and personal life when using social networking websites. Commonly reported unprofessional postings include: violations of patient confidentiality; learners' use of profanity; discriminatory language; depiction of intoxication; and sexually suggestive material (Ly, 2010; Chretien et al., 2009).

## Assessment

Assessment is a central component in the overall quality of teaching and learning in HE and should be viewed positively as an opportunity for you to demonstrate your knowledge. ODP courses may vary in how they assess academic and clinical skills. Most will use a mixed economy of assessment methods to capture an all-round, holistic view of a learner's competence and performance. Assessment, whether formative or summative in nature, sets clear expectations, establishes a reasonable workload for learners and provides opportunities for you to self-monitor, practise and receive feedback. Assessment is an integral component of a coherent educational experience.

It is well documented that learners value, and expect, transparency in the way their knowledge will be assessed. There needs to be a clear relationship between lectures, tutorials, clinical practice and subject resources and what they are expected to demonstrate in any assessment method. Assessment is about making a decision on the present position of the learner's learning and therefore should be seen as a chance to consolidate your knowledge and understanding, in addition to demonstrating to your tutors, mentors, patients and yourself what you know (Burns and Sinfield, 2012). Assessment can provide effective feedback about the grades they have achieved; it rewards their efforts and achievements and offers suggestions for how they can improve their all-round performances.

### Formative assessment

Generally, formative assessment is designed to help tutor/mentor identify the learner's strength and weaknesses, through rich conversations that continually build and go deeper. It provides effective, timely feedback to enable learners to advance their learning, therefore actively involving learners in their own learning. Ultimately, formative assessment nurtures the concept of increased autonomy and responsibility for learning in the learner (Andrade and Cizek, 2010). The educational objective is to move the learner from passive receiver of information to a self-reliant thinker (CODP, 2011).

There are a number of methods that could be used in formative assessment, for example, the use of a logbook to record the number of orthopaedic cases you have scrubbed for could provide evidence of consistent practice. In more complex practice, the use of high-fidelity simulation has enabled skills to be practised formatively in a safe environment and constructively built upon before any holistic summative assessment. In an academic example, an online quiz set by a tutor, a low score in pharmacology topics may indicate that there is a need to review the revision strategy or how the subject has to be learned. Both these examples identify the strength and weaknesses and with feedback enable learners to advance their learning in preparation for summative assessment.

## Summative assessment

Summative assessment is comprehensive in nature, provides accountability and is used to check the level of learning and experiences that have met the learning outcomes. Summative assessment is constructively aligned to reflect the learning outcomes (Burns and Sinfield, 2012); for example, if upon completion of a module you will have the knowledge and understanding to pass an exam, taking the exam would be summative in nature since it is based on the cumulative learning experience of the module. Summative assessments address the same domains, concepts and skills as formative assessments. They do not include anything new or unfamiliar to learners, the assessment has to be fair and valid (Cassidy, 2009). Common summative assessment methods used in operating department practice education include: assignments; examinations; presentations; and the achievement of prescribed clinical practice outcomes.

It is important that an ODP learner understands the expected performance criteria (grading) in any summative assessment as using the grades and the descriptor of the grades in formative assessment is a useful strategy in preparing for summative assessment. The ODP learner can then use these rubrics to self-assess their work formatively before final submission to identify their academic strengths and weaknesses formatively.

Fotheringham (2010) provided a practical insight into the concept of 'triangulation' to support the use of multiple assessment tools. Use different methods to provide a holistic view of the academic performances, clinical skills and professionalism of the learner across the psychomotor, cognitive and professional domains (Gillespie and Hamlin, 2009). Mentors consider technical and procedural knowledge as fundamental to clinical competence but it must be acknowledged that communication, teamwork and co-ordinating the clinical workload are important concepts that have to be included in the assessment process (Gillespie et al., 2009).

## Simulation

With an increase in concerns for patient safety and the need to reduce critical errors in practice, ODP education continues to strive to develop competent and confident learners through formative learning experiences. Coupled with an increased knowledge of medical science, new treatments and complex healthcare systems, ODPs need the capability to analyse a patient's clinical condition and respond accordingly to implement safe and effective care (Reid-Searle et al., 2011). Consequently, the use of simulation, either formative or summative in nature, has evolved over the last 50 years from simple part-task training devices to complex manikins capable of imitating a variety of clinical situations (Harper and Eales-Reynolds, 2011). Recent studies show that the use of simulation in an interprofessional context promotes a sustained positive effect on learner's attitudes to learning and teamworking (Buckley et al., 2012; Reid-Searle et al., 2011).

Simulation can appeal to most learning styles as it enhances the cognition and psychomotor skills required to understand the clinical situation and the bigger concepts around collaborative working (Buckley et al., 2012; Harper and Eales-Reynolds, 2011). Different complex situations can be created and analysed, but in a safe learning environment promoting deeper reflective learning and confidence to transfer new skills to the reality of clinical practice (Harper and Eales-Reynolds, 2011).

### Grading competence

Perioperative competence is an eclectic concept that has been difficult to define and even more difficult to measure. Competence has been described in relation to standards of practice with little emphasis placed on its interpersonal aspects. Cassidy (2009) suggests that competence is something that someone has learned giving them 'specialized' knowledge characterized by familiarity with perioperative practice guidelines and standards of care, and the human factors of interpersonal and social aspects of team interactions. However, there is no clear consensus on competence; furthermore, assessing a learner as competent may be complicated by the assessors' subjective interpretations of the assessment criteria (Cassidy, 2009). Most literature on the subject of clinical competence advocates the use of rubrics or indicators to assist with consistent assessment and evaluation of performance. Rubrics provide specific descriptions of the responses for each criteria and match proficiency levels and quality ratings. They precisely pinpoint what constituted the decision for the grade/scale.

Competence grading scales and modified versions are often used in the assessment of clinical practice. Here we reiterate the importance of formative assessment and effective, timely feedback (Juwah et al., 2004; Lennie and Juwah, 2010). If both learner and mentor use a scale, strength and weaknesses across the practice domains can be identified and further developed to meet the required grade. When learners engage with feedback, verbal or written through reflective practice, new personal learning objectives can be set. If a learner failed a clinical practice assessment, understanding the indicators of the scale will identify the criteria for development but also provides justification for such an assessment decision for the mentor (Duffy, 2003). The mentor is seen as the 'gatekeeper' to the profession and has the professional responsibility of inferring competence on the learner, a decision that needs to be free from subjectivity (CODP, 2009).

The issue of subjectivity and valid assessment for mentors contributes to the difficulties that mentors have in failing a learner in clinical practice; in some cases they 'fail to fail' (Duffy, 2003). The language used in assessment tools is an important factor in enabling the mentor and learner to interpret competence (Gillespie et al., 2009). Competence assessment is affected by many situational factors and Yanhua and Watson (2011) argue that these can detract from a valid reliable measurement of the competence level of the learner. Furthermore, the clinical competence of newly registered staff has become a crucial issue related to profession standards and public safety (Darzi, 2008)

Professional behaviours and appropriate skills on the part of individual practitioners are the overwhelmingly prevalent factors that led to the Mid Staffordshire NHS Foundation Trust Inquiry (Francis, 2012). These professional values are central to the delivery of high-quality healthcare education and therefore mentors have a duty of care to the public through their registration to ensure that learners develop into practitioners fit for purpose, practice and their award.

### Portfolios

The use of portfolios is recognized as a valuable tool for the collection of evidence towards the assessment of the domains of practice (McCoglan, 2008) and should provide evidence of learning experiences and achievements in both academic and practice settings (Lewis, 2010; Karsten, 2012). Current ODP learners will generally have a practice portfolio that will contain, for example, academic achievements, practice outcomes, practice experiences, reflection and case studies, thus preparing the ODP learner to maintain their evidence of professional development throughout their career. As information technology tools are developed and introduced into the everyday life at university, it is important that the learner embraces the concept of ePortfolios in order to demonstrate academic achievement, clinical competence and critical thinking through this innovative and technically advanced method (Jisc, 2008; Lewis, 2010; Karsten, 2012).

## Learning support

Universities in England and Wales have a 'duty to make reasonable adjustments' for learners with disabilities, and this includes learners with dyslexia or other specific learning needs. This duty of care ensures that individuals are not discriminated against in relationship to 'the arrangements made for deciding upon whom to confer a qualification' under the Equality Act 2010 (HM Government, 2010: ch. 15).

Education providers have a duty to find out how they can make 'reasonable adjustments' to meet the needs of learners with disabilities. Whether or not an adjustment is reasonable depends on many factors such as the cost of the adjustment not just financial but logistical and the effect of the adjustment.

The intensity of ODP courses means that early diagnosis of learning disabilities is beneficial and early access to screening of learners is common to ensure that individuals are supported throughout their studies (Wray et al., 2008).

## Conclusion

The skills, practices and attitudes fundamental to the ODP are gained from the whole of the educational experience. The information within this chapter has provided a perceptive insight for both new learners and those practitioners returning to learning into the teaching, learning and assessment approaches used in the HE setting. It is hoped that the applied exploration of the topics will contribute to a successful educational experience and promote the reader to become an autonomous, self-directed learner who is proficient in delivering evidence-based, individualized, high-quality patient care. Ultimately, developing your learning throughout your career as an ODP contributes to the development of an accountable and responsible practitioner who is fit for purpose, practice and award.

### Key points

- Understanding your learning style can successfully guide your learning.
- Understanding educational theories helps to promote self-directed, self-reliant and effective learning.
- Use formative assessment as a directive feedback to identify learning needs.
- Grading scales provide useful feedback and justifies assessment decisions.
- Portfolios are valuable tools for the collection of evidence for the assessment of the practice and learning development.
- There are specific support mechanisms available for individuals with specific learning disabilities.

### References and further reading

Andrade, H.L. and Cizek, G.J. (2010) *Handbook of Formative Assessment*. London: Routledge.

Bloom, B. (1994) *Reflections on the Development and Use of the Taxonomy*, in Anderson, Lorin W. and Sosniak, Lauren A. (eds) (1994) *Bloom's Taxonomy: A Forty-year Retrospective*. Chicago, IL: National Society for the Study of Education.

Booth, H. cited in Ly, K. (2010) 'Social networking: blurring the personal and professional', *Technic: The Journal of Operating Department Practice*, 1 (18): 2–3.

Buckley, S., Hensman, M., Thomas, S., Dudley, R., Nevin, G. and Cleman, J. (2012) 'Developing interprofessional simulation in the undergraduate setting: experience with five different professional groups', *Journal of Interprofessional Care*, 26: 362–69.

Burns, T. and Sinfield, S. (2012) *Essential Study Skills: The Complete Guide to Success at University* (3rd edn.). London: Sage Publications.

Cassidy, S. (2009) 'Interpretation of competence in learner assessment', *Nursing Standard*, 23 (18): 39–46.

Chretien, K.C., Grevsen, S.R., Chretien, J.P. and Kind, T. (2009) 'Online posting of unprofessional content by medical students', *Journal of the American Medical Association*, 302 (12): 1309–15 (doi: 10.1001/jama.2009.1387).

College of Operating Department Practitioners (CODP) (2009) *Standards, Recommendations and Guidance for Mentors and Practice Placements: Supporting Pre-registration Education in Operating Department Practice*. London: CODP.

College of Operating Department Practitioners (CODP) (2011) *Bachelor of Science (Hons) in Operating Department Practice – England, Northern Ireland and Wales: Curriculum Document*. London: CODP.

D'Amore, A., James, S. and Mitchell, E.K.L. (2011) 'Learning styles of first-year undergraduate nursing and midwifery students: a cross-sectional survey utilising the Kolb Learning Style Inventory', *Nurse Education Today*, 32: 506–15.

Darzi, A. (2008) *High Quality Care for All: NHS Next Stage Review Final Report*. London: Department of Health (DH), CM 7432.

Duffy, K. (2003) *Failing Students: A Qualitative Study of Factors that Influence the Decisions Regarding the Assessment of Students' Competence to Practice*. Glasgow: Caledonian Nursing and Midwifery Research Centre, Glasgow Caledonian University.

Fleming, N.D. (2012) *VARK: A Guide to Learning Styles*. Available online at http://www.varklearn.com/english/page.asp?pquestionnaire (accessed 15 January 2013).

Fotheringham, D. (2010) 'Triangulation for the assessment of clinical nursing skills: a review of theory, use and methodology', *International Journal of Nursing Studies*, 47 (3): 386–91.

Francis, R. (2010) *Report into Mid-Staffordshire NHS Foundation Trust*. Available online at http://www.dh.gov.uk/en/Publicationsandstatistics/Publications/PublicationsPolicyAndGuidance/DH_113018 (accessed 15 January 2013).

Gillespie, B.M. and Hamlin, L. (2009) 'A synthesis of the literature on "competence" as it applies to perioperative nursing', *Association of Perioperative Registered Nurses*, 90 (2): 245–58.

Gillespie, B.M., Chaboyer, Wallis, M., W., Chang, H-Y.A. and Werder, H. (2009) 'Operating theatre nurses' perceptions of competence: a focus group study', *Journal of Advanced Nursing*, 65 (5): 90–101.

Harper, M. and Eales-Reynolds, L.J. (2011) 'Simulation: knowledge transfer from classroom to patient care', *Technic: The Journal of Operating Department Practice*, 2 (4): 12–15.

Health and Care Professions Council (HCPC) (2012) *Standards of Education and Training*. London: HCPC.

Higher Education Academy (HEA) (2011) *Deep and Surface Approaches to Learning*. Available online at http://84.22.166.132/learning-and-teaching-theory-guide/deep-and-surface-approaches-learning.html (accessed 15 January 2013).

HM Government (2010) *Equality Act 2010*. London: Stationery Office.

Horton, D., Wiederman, S. and Saint, D. (2012) 'Assessment outcome is weakly correlated with lecture attendance: influence of learning style and use of alternative materials', *Advances in Physiology Education*, 36 (2): 108–15.

Hutchinson, L. (2007) *Teaching and Learning in the Clinical Context*. Available online at http://www.faculty.londondeanery.ac.uk/e-learning/assessing-educational-needs/Teaching_learning_in_clinical_context.pdf (accessed 15 January 2013).

Joint Information Systems Committee (JISC) (2008) *Effective Practice with e-Portfolios*. Bristol: JISC infoNet.

Joint Information Systems Committee (JISC) (2010) *Recording Lectures: Legal Considerations*. Bristol: JISC Legal Information.

Juwah, C., Macfarlane-Dick, D., Matthew, B., Nicol, D., Ross, D. and Smith, B. (2004) *Enhancing Student Learning through Effective Formative Feedback*. York: HEA Generic Centre.

Karsten, K. (2012) 'Using ePortfolio to demonstrate competence in associate degree nursing learners', *Teaching and Learning in Nursing*, 7: 23–26.

Kolb, D.A. (1984) *Experiential Learning Experience as a Source of Learning and Development*. Upper Saddle River, NJ: Prentice Hall.

Lennie, S.C. and Juwah, C. (2010) 'Exploring assessment for learning during dietetic practice placements', *Journal of Human Nutrition and Dietetics*, 23: 217–23.

Lewis, T. (2010) 'Working measures: online clinical practice assessment', *Technic: The Journal of Operating Department Practice*, 1 (2): 15.

Ly, K. (2010) 'Social networking: blurring the personal and professional', *Technic: The Journal of Operating Department Practice*, 1 (18): 2–3.

McColgan, K. (2008) 'The value of portfolio building and the registered nurse: a review of the literature, Karen McColgan explores the value of portfolio building', *Journal of Perioperative Practice*, 18 (2): 64–69.

Mobbs, R. (2012) *Bloom's Taxonomy*. Available online at ttp://www2.le.ac.uk/departments/gradschool/training/resources/teaching/theories/bloom?searchterm=bloom, (accessed 15 January 2013).

National Archives (2013) *Data Protection Act 1998*. Available online at http://www.legislation.gov.uk/ukpga/1998/29/contents (accessed 2 May 2013).

Nikoi, S. (2008) *Work-based Learners in Further Education* (WoLF) project. Leicester: University of Leicester.

Nursing and Midwifery Council and General Medical Council (2012) *Joint Statement on Professional Values*. Available online at http://www.nmc-uk.org/Press-and-media/Latest-news/NMC-and-GMC-release-joint-statement-on-professional-values/ (accessed 15 January 2013).

Open University (2011) *Using Mobile Devices*. Available online at http://www.open.ac.uk/pc4study/toptips/using-gadgets.php, (accessed 16 January 2013).

Quality Assurance Agency (QAA) for Higher Education (2007) *Outcomes from Institutional Audit: The Adoption and Use of LEARNING Outcomes*. Gloucester: QAA.

Quality Assurance Agency (QAA) for Higher Education (2012) *Assuring Standards and Quality*. Available online at http://www.qaa.ac.uk/AssuringStandardsAndQuality/Pages/default.aspx (accessed 15 January 2013).

Reid-Searle, K., Eaton, A., Vieth, L. and Happell, B. (2011) 'The educator inside the patient: learner's insight into the use of high fidelity silicone patient simulation', *Journal of Clinical Nursing*, 20: 2752–60.

Richardson, J.T.E. (2011) 'Approaches to studying, conceptions of learning and learning styles in HE', *Learning and Individual Differences*, 21: 288–93.

Sarafino, E.P. (2008) *Health Psychology: Biopsychosocial Interactions*. Hoboken, NJ: John Wiley & Sons, Inc.

Smith, K. (2008) *Howard Gardner, Multiple Intelligences and Education*. Available online at http://www.infed.org/thinkers/gardner.htm (accessed 15 January 2013).

University of Dublin (2011) *Using Biggs' Model of Constructive Alignment in Curriculum Design*. Available online at http://www.ucdoer.ie/index.php/Using_Biggs'_Model_of_Constructive_ Alignment_in_Curriculum_Design/Introduction (accessed 15 January 2013).

Wray, J., Harrison, P., Aspland, J., Taghzouit, J., Pace, K. and Gibson H. (2008) *The Impact of Specific Learning Difficulties (SpLD) on the Progression and Retention of Learner Nurses*. Hull: University of Hull.

Yanhua, C. and Watson, R. (2011) 'A review of clinical competence assessment in nursing', *Nurse Education Today*, 31 (8): 832–36.

Yudkowsky, R., Downing, S.M. and Scott Wirth, S. (2008) 'Simpler standards for local performance examinations: the yes/no Angoff and whole-test Ebel', *Teaching and Learning in Medicine: An International Journal*, 20 (3): 212–17.

# 3 Research and evidence-based practice for operating department practice

## Hannah Abbott

**Key topics**

- Origin and development of professional knowledge
- Evidence-based practice
- Research
- Research ethics
- Paradigms of research

- Quantitative research
- Qualitative research
- Mixed-methods research
- Literature review
- Critical appraisal of literature
- Clinical audit

## Introduction

Research impacts and underpins almost everything we do in both our professional and personal lives and we frequently engage with some form of research; for example, the completion of surveys. In our professional lives as Operating Department Practitioners (ODPs) we use research evidence to develop our knowledge and enhance our practice and therefore it is important to understand how this knowledge is generated so that published papers can be used effectively. This chapter therefore explores the philosophy that underpins research and the methodologies that may be employed within healthcare research. Research is an extensive topic and there are many texts that focus on just one aspect of research and consequently it is not possible to cover all aspects in depth within the scope of this chapter. What this chapter aims to provide therefore is a good overview of the principles of research and clinical audit that will give you the skills to be able to read and appraise a paper effectively thus enabling you to utilize research in your career as an ODP. In addition, this chapter also aims to demonstrate that research is integral to the professional role and hence to give you the confidence to consider your own research interests and how you may further develop these.

## Why is this relevant?

There have been many different national publications relating to numerous aspects of healthcare delivery. However, all of these have one key theme – the delivery of high-quality patient care; the responsibility to deliver this care is shared by all practitioners including ODPs. As ODPs, therefore, how do we know that we are delivering high-quality care to every patient and that we are instilling this culture within our professional practice? Ultimately, we all have to start with our own individual practice and ODPs must 'be able to assure the quality of their practice' (Health and Care Professions

Council (HCPC), 2014, Standard 12) that includes engaging in evidence-based practice, systematic evaluation of practice, participation in audit and the utilization of qualitative and quantitative data (HCPC, 2014). It is therefore impossible for an ODP to deliver high-quality care and meet the threshold standards for professional registration without engaging with research.

The perioperative environment is a dynamic environment that is continually evolving to meet increasingly complex needs; this may be the patient needs and the complexity of the co-morbidities, it may be the delivery of anaesthesia, or complex surgical procedures and equipment. Whatever the nature of the complexity, the knowledge and skill set of ODPs must advance to meet these needs and therefore ODPs need to engage with research as part of their professional responsibility: 'you must keep your professional knowledge and skills up to date' (HCPC, 2012: 10). This may be achieved in a number of ways as part of continued professional development (CPD), which is discussed in more detail in Chapter 11. However, it is not possible to ensure our knowledge is current without ever reading the new developments and research papers published in a range of journals and accessible via a National Health Service (NHS) Athens account or university databases. This chapter therefore supports you in engagement with research for the provision of high-quality care and your own development as a professional.

## The origin and development of professional knowledge

Think about our professional practice for a moment – why do we do things in the way we do; for example, why do you lay your scrub trolley in a certain way? Maybe it is because it is how you have always done it, or maybe it is how you were taught by your mentor, or maybe it is the '. . . hospital way'; a lot of the skills we learn were taught by mentors who were taught by mentors before them but how did that knowledge originate and how did it evolve?

As we have already mentioned, some of the operating department practice has been passed from ODP to student over the years through teaching and observation of practice and via textbooks; this is termed as 'traditional knowledge' that is considered important in both the sharing of knowledge and in the development of professional identity (Parahoo, 2006). Some of these traditional practices become rituals that are performed without thinking about it in an analytical way but rather as they have always been done (Courtney et al., 2010) and it has been suggested that ritualistic practice helps practitioners and patients manage the emotional and social interactions within the role (Strange, 2001). It is not however acceptable to simply undertake tasks automatically without ever questioning practice; this is not to say that some of these traditional practices are sub-optimal, it may be that it remains the best approach, but in order to validate this we must question and explore evidence.

Professional knowledge has also evolved through experience and reflective practice (Chapter 8) and the results of this experiential learning can be shared to enhance the learning experiences of others. While experiential learning is valuable within perioperative practice, it is important that ODPs recognize that this knowledge will be limited by their own experiences and must therefore be aware that relying purely on experiential knowledge can actually restrict their professional development. For example, an ODP working with paediatric patients may feel that one distraction technique is preferable for cannulation as this has always worked effectively for them and their colleagues in the past. However, this historic local practice may actually restrict further development as ODPs may not be willing to explore new techniques which may improve current practice. Linked to experiential learning is the consideration of intuition as a source of knowledge. However, this is difficult to define and cannot be the topic of empirical research (Parahoo, 2006), but despite this many ODPs may report having 'a feeling' that something is wrong or requires further investigation. It may be argued however that this is not attributed to intuition but rather to a combination of clinical knowledge, experience and systematic patient assessment that allows a practitioner to rapidly assimilate information regarding the patient and make a prompt decision regarding the plan of care.

The development of professional knowledge is ever evolving and while some of our current practices may be attributed to tradition, ritual or experiential learning, this is clearly not sufficient for the continued provision of high-quality care. This is not to suggest that current perioperative practice is poor; rather, it should be questioned to ensure that it is the best current practice and based on robust evidence.

**Stop and think**

If someone questioned your practice and asked "why do you do that?" what would you say?

Would you be able to refer to literature? Could you explain the alternative methods and justify why yours is best overall?

For example, if someone asked you: 'Why do you assist with rapid sequence induction in that way?' How would you answer – because it was the way you were taught? Or because that is what that individual anaesthetist likes? Or would you be able to critically discuss the literature regarding the efficacy of cricoid pressure, the amount of pressure and the timing of application?

Remember that registered ODPs must 'be able to practise as an autonomous professional' (HCPC 2014, Standard 4) and this requires that the ODP is able to justify their decisions.

## Evidence-based practice

In this chapter we have already considered the evolution of our professional knowledge and you have considered why you need to be able to provide a rationale for your practice, based upon evidence and this leads into the principle of evidence-based practice. There are a number of misconceptions about evidence-based practice, often that by following the recommendations of one published paper the ODP is implementing evidence-based practice.

Evidence-based practice however is not basing your practice upon one research paper nor is it practising in a traditional, ritualistic way because this is how you were taught some time ago (Prasun, 2013). The term 'evidence-based practice' demonstrates a focus on empirical evidence about what is effective in practice (Glasziou et al., 2003) and therefore evidence-based practice integrates research evidence with clinical experience and knowledge about the patient or procedure, in the context of the patient's own preferences and values (Sackett et al., 2001). The ODP therefore needs to be able to assimilate all their knowledge related to the case and use this to inform their practice accordingly; for example, the ODP may consider the empirical knowledge about the benefits and limitations of spinal anaesthesia in conjunction with the knowledge they gained from a qualitative paper about the patient experience and use this along with their own clinical experience and assessment of the patient to deliver an evidence-based plan of care to the perioperative patient.

Evidence-based practice is implemented on a larger scale through the development of evidence-based practice guidelines that are developed through synthesizing the evidence and considering the validity of this in order to make recommendations for practice (Beyea, 2004). It is considered that the subsequent implementation of evidence-based practice guidelines should reduce variability and result in an overall improvement in patient care (Beyea, 2004). This is why it is important for clinical guidelines to be reviewed on a regular basis as new research findings may require guidelines to be updated to ensure practice continues to reflect the most current, valid evidence base.

## Research

Research is a systematic process that generates new knowledge to contribute to the wider body of knowledge. The 'body of knowledge' is a term, which is used frequently to describe the unique knowledge about a specific topic area, and hence the operating department practice body of knowledge includes clinical practice in addition to knowledge about the specific education of ODPs. As a relatively new profession, the ODP specific body of knowledge is evolving as more practitioners undertake research and publish their findings in professional journals. However, our body of knowledge will overlap with the body of knowledge of associated professions within the perioperative environment.

There are a number of differing views regarding the purpose and application of research. The scientific view of research is that it is purely the discovery of knowledge that is important rather than the application of this knowledge and hence it has been argued that researchers are not responsible for the impact or application of their research. Many ODPs and other healthcare practitioners may find that this scientific view conflicts with their professional obligations that their activities should benefit the patient. There is however also the view that those who fund research have an influence on the objectives and potential application of the study; in the case of publicly funded research it has been suggested that the public (our potential patients) have a role in the identification of research priorities. If we consider research in the context of the perioperative environment, therefore, it would seem crucial that this research was relevant to the service provided and would have some benefit to our patients; hence, while healthcare research does contribute to the body of knowledge, it is also designed to make a contribution to professional practice.

### Aims, questions and hypothesis

All research projects will have a clear focus; however, depending on the topic and approach, this can be expressed in a number of different ways – as an aim, a question or a hypothesis. However, it is important to note at this point that while a researcher will establish this early in their research, it may not be explicitly stated in the published paper, but it will be evident from the title and introduction.

Setting an aim for a research project allows the researcher to express a statement of their intent and provides a focus for the study and this approach may be often used in qualitative research that takes a more reflexive approach. When framing the research question using an aim, it must be possible to achieve this within the study; for example, 'this study aims to determine the patient's lived experience of day surgery'.

Framing the study topic as a question is a common approach and can be used effectively for both quantitative and qualitative primary research, and for literature review projects. The use of a question is particularly useful for new researchers as it provides a clear focus as the study must answer the question. In healthcare research a PICO framework is often used to define the question and this considers the population, intervention, comparison and outcome; for example, 'Does total intravenous anaesthesia (intervention) reduce the incidence of post-operative nausea and vomiting (PONV) (outcome) when compared with sevoflurane (comparison) in adult patients undergoing gynaecology surgery (population)'. Using this framework therefore can be helpful to refine an initial research idea into a clearly focused question as it allows the ODP to narrow the focus of their study and this process encourages the consideration of variables that can impact results and how they can be reduced by clearly focusing the population. The PICO framework is frequently used to frame the question for literature reviews and this process can then be used to support the identification of search terms, as multiple terms can be identified under each section. There are limitations to this tool however as in some studies (particularly qualitative) there may not be a defined outcome or in others there may not be a comparison and therefore while the principles may be helpful, it is important that PICO is used as an enabling tool rather than a restrictive one.

Hypotheses are commonly employed in quantitative studies and form a key component of statistical analysis. A hypothesis is simply an educated prediction of the expected findings; this may result from previous studies or a review of the literature. The key to using a hypothesis to express the study focus is that the hypothesis must be testable and the study will seek to prove or disprove the overarching hypothesis; consequently, this is the usual approach for scientific, experimental studies. In quantitative research, inferential statistical tests are performed under the null hypothesis that are discussed later in the chapter.

## Research ethics

This chapter has shown that research is pivotal to the continued development of perioperative care. However, there can be an element of risk associated with research and this may be either physiological or psychological, and therefore it is essential that there is a robust research governance system to ensure quality in health and social care (Department of Health (DH), 2005). Research ethics are a complex topic and the underpinning principles are explored in more detail in Chapter 7; this chapter therefore aims to provide the reader with an overview of the practical considerations regarding research ethics. The primary consideration of any research must be the protection of the participants' dignity, rights, safety and wellbeing and consequently informed consent is central to ethical research (DH, 2005). To ensure informed consent has been obtained all potential participants must be fully informed about the risks, benefits and potential discomfort related to participation in addition to the aims of the study, the methodology and the sources of funding and their right to withdraw at any time. It has been shown that patient satisfaction with study information could be improved (Länsimies-Antikainen et al., 2009) and hence it is good practice for participants to be provided with written information as a point of reference; this may be at the pre-assessment so that a patient has sufficient time to consider participation prior to their surgery.

In the UK ethical approval for healthcare research is via the National Research Ethics Service (NRES), which aims to protect the interests of research participants and to facilitate ethical research that has benefits to both the participants and the wider community (Health Research Authority, 2013). This is achieved by the approval of research by Research Ethics Committees (RECs) that are independent panels that review applications and decide whether the proposed research is ethical (Health Research Authority, 2013); further information about the application process can be found on their website. It is essential therefore that ethical approval is obtained prior to the commencement of the data collection and consequently the time to complete this process must be factored into any work plan. In the case of research that is undertaken as part of a university programme of study and does not involve data collection in a hospital, for example a project to determine the knowledge other healthcare students have of the ODP role, ethical approval must be obtained from the university ethics committee. In addition to gaining ethical approval, appropriate access permissions must be sought from the individual responsible for the 'care' of the participants; it is not appropriate to collect data from any participants without this approval.

## Paradigms of research

A paradigm is essentially a philosophical belief system and in the context of research this is the fundamental belief regarding the production of knowledge. In research there are two differing belief systems regarding the generation of knowledge and these translate into two approaches to research – quantitative and qualitative. It is often assumed that these two paradigms are defined by the variable measured and whether this is a quantity or a quality; this is not the case however as it is the underpinning philosophy that defines the methodology. It is therefore possible to measure a quality, for example feelings of satisfaction, but using a quantitative approach that results in numerical data for analysis.

The positivist paradigm believes that objective knowledge can be produced by employing a rigorous methodology (Broom and Willis, 2007) and employs a scientific method of testing hypothesis and using a reductionist approach to reduce phenomena to statements of law based upon the probability of occurrence (Parahoo, 2006). This positivist approach therefore underpins quantitative research that uses scientific principles to produce firm conclusions and 'rules' relating to perioperative care that can be generalized to the wider population; for example, the efficacy of different anaesthetic agents.

Interpretivism is a direct contrast to positivism and adopts the view that knowledge is a social construct and therefore to understand human behaviour it must be explored within the context in which it occurs (Parahoo, 2006). This philosophical approach therefore underpins the qualitative approach that explores the lived human experiences and behaviours within specific settings and hence offers greater depth but cannot be generalized in the same way as quantitative research. Therefore using this approach, for example, to explore ODP students' experiences of their clinical placements, would produce results that were specific to the hospital placement (context) and may not be generalized to all ODP students who would undertake placements in different contexts, for example more specialized hospitals.

## Quantitative research

Quantitative research uses numerical analysis to examine the relationship between measured variables; for example, the ODP may use this approach to determine if there is a relationship between duration of the anaesthetic and the length of time spent in the post-anaesthetic care unit. Quantitative research therefore can provide important information that will directly impact the care of the patient; for example, the efficacy of a procedure when compared with an alternative or the incidence of side-effects of a particular drug. Consequently, these findings can have a direct impact upon the care of the perioperative patient and the provision of services within a department.

### Methods

There are a number of different quantitative methodologies that may be employed to address the research question; however, these can generally be described as one of three different designs – experimental, survey and case study:

- Experimental research designs aim to determine relationships between variables and a range of experimental methodologies may be employed to determine these. The randomized control study (RCT) is considered the most robust methodology as it randomly assigns participants to an intervention and a control group and compares the effect of the intervention upon the two groups. The RCT approach is generally used when trialling a new intervention and therefore while ODPs will read a number of RCT studies to develop their knowledge, it is less likely an ODP would be the sole investigator on an RCT project. Quasi-experimental studies also compare the effect of an intervention against a control group. However, participants are allocated rather than randomized into the two groups; this approach also includes before and after studies that are frequently used to measure the efficacy of healthcare interventions (Centre for Reviews and Dissemination (CRD), 2009). ODPs will find a number of experimental studies to support their practice, particularly relating to the efficacy or side-effects of different drug regimes and therefore it is important that ODPs become familiar with this approach in order to critique articles effectively.

- Survey research designs are utilized to collect a large amount of information from a population and this approach is commonly employed by ODPs conducting research to improve practice within the perioperative environment. This approach can collect information regarding the incidence, frequency, severity and distribution of variables within a population; this can then be used to identify relationships within the data. For example this approach would have been used to identify risk factors for PONV by surveying the patients who experience this, the nature of their surgery, their age and gender.
- Case studies are focused on specific situations and collect a range of information pertinent to the given situation; this data will be predominantly descriptive although the researcher will explore any relationship between variables (Parahoo, 2006). The ODP may therefore use this approach at a local or national level to explore a specific adverse incident, for example difficult airways.

These are the frequently employed approaches to research design; however, there are a number of specific methodologies within these categories and there is also some potential for methodologies to be adapted to fit specific topics. When undertaking research as part of an academic award this is something that you would discuss with your supervisor.


### Blinding

Blinding may be utilized in quantitative studies to minimize the risk of observer bias as theoretically if either the participant or the observer knows their group allocation it may impact upon their responses in the study. There are two types of blinding:

- Single blind studies where either participant or researcher (not both) is blinded to the group allocation. In single blind studies it is generally the participant who is blind to the group allocation; for example, a patient may not know which anaesthetic maintenance agent they are receiving.
- Double blind studies where both the participant and the researcher are blinded to the group allocation.

When you read papers the methodology will include blinding and how this was achieved; it is important to then consider how important blinding is to the results; for example, objective physiological measurements will not be affected by knowledge of group allocation. Any safety considerations of blinding must be considered; for example, if the patient and/or researcher do not know the nature of the medication administered. In addition, there are potentially ethical issues related to blinding; for example, when 'sham surgery' is used for the control group it may be considered whether it is ethical to subject participants to an unnecessary anaesthetic (Katz, 2006).


### Sampling

When collecting data for qualitative studies, ideally the ODP researcher would like to collect data from everyone in the relevant population. However, this is not feasible and therefore it is necessary to collect data from a sample of the study population. There are a number of different sampling methods that are commonly employed in quantitative research. These are generally probability samples that are randomized, for example, through computer-generated random numbers or random number tables. There are also non-probability sampling methods that may occasionally be employed; for example, accidental or volunteer sampling, which are samples of convenience. These approaches however do not have the same rigour as randomized techniques as not all members of the potential population have an equal chance of being selected, hence bias can be introduced at this stage of the study. For example, if you wanted to discover what the public knowledge of the ODP role was you could survey passers-by in the town centre one weekday. However, this would exclude a large proportion of the working population and thus introduce bias. It is important that the ODP undertaking research therefore considers how they will identify their sample and it is useful to read a number of papers to see what methods other researchers have used effectively to collect data within the perioperative environment.

The sample size is also central to quantitative studies as the sample must be sufficient to detect any significant differences; however, it is not appropriate to collect excessive, unnecessary data. The sample size is generally determined by a power analysis; this calculation considers the magnitude of the expected difference due to the intervention and will calculate the number of participants required to show a statistically significant difference if one exists. If the expected difference is small then a larger sample size will be required to show any significant differences. It should be remembered that some studies will conduct their power analysis based upon the primary outcome and therefore may be underpowered for the secondary outcomes. The ODP should therefore consider the sample size and also consider this in the context of their clinical knowledge to make an assessment of adequacy of sample size and the feasibility of collecting data in the given time.

### Data collection

Quantitative data can be collected in a number of ways to meet the aims of the study and this frequently involves collecting experimental data or physiological measurements. Many quantitative studies that aim to gain information regarding the patient experience will use surveys, which may include simple 'yes or no' questions or more complex scales to grade information. Many ODPs use surveys in their research as these are an effective way of gathering a large amount of data. However, the response rates tend to be low and therefore a significant number of questionnaires need to be distributed to elicit the required number of responses. The development of surveys is a complex process and hence sufficient time must be allocated for this process and to test the survey instrument for construct validity, which is to test that the survey measures what it is intended to measure.

### Data analysis and statistics – some simplification and reduction

Statistical analysis of data is a feature of quantitative research studies and can be found in the results section of a published paper. There are two types of statistical analysis: descriptive statistics and inferential statistics and it is important for ODPs to have an appreciation of both of these to be able to appraise a paper critically and effectively.

Descriptive statistics will feature in all quantitative papers and will also be used in reporting clinical audit results. These serve to summarize and describe the data using simple mathematic measurements; for example, the mean value, the range and percentages. This allows you to compare the two sample groups, for example you may read that there is a higher incidence of anti-emetic therapy following isoflurane maintenance (38.1 per cent) when compared with propofol (11.9 per cent) (Gecaj-Gashi et al., 2010). While you can therefore see any observed difference between the two groups, you may also want to know if this difference is due to a true difference resulting from the interventions or whether it may have occurred by chance, and this is where inferential statistics are beneficial.

Inferential statistics also feature in the majority of quantitative research papers but are not generally used in clinical audit; these statistics are used to determine whether the observed relationship is greater than that which would be expected by chance and hence whether it is a true relationship between the two variables or whether it has occurred by chance (Katz, 2006). There are a number of statistical tests that can be performed (Table 3.1) on the data and these depend on whether the test aims to determine difference or correlation and whether the data is parametric or not; parametric data is normally distributed and hence most biological measurements result in normally distributed data. This table is designed to serve as a point of reference when reading published papers and

**Table 3.1** A summary of commonly used statistical tests

| Statistical test | Tests for . . . | Data must be . . . |
|---|---|---|
| t-test | Differences between two population means | Parametric |
| Mann–Whitney U Test | Differences between two population medians | Non-parametric |
| Wilcoxon Matched Pairs (Signed Rank) Test | Differences between population medians of two matched samples | Non-parametric |
| Analysis of Variance (ANOVA) | Difference in population means of more than two populations | Parametric |
| Kruskal Wallis Test | Difference in medians of three or more populations | Parametric |
| Pearson Correlation Coefficient | Correlation between two data sets | Parametric |
| Spearman Rank Correlation Coefficient | Correlation between two sets of measurements | Non-parametric |
| Chi Squared Test | Association between two variables | Non-parametric |

conducting critical appraisal, as this process asks you to consider the suitability of the statistical tests employed.

All these statistical tests are performed under what is known as the 'null hypothesis' that means there is no difference/correlation/association (as appropriate to the test) between the two (or more) variables; the statistical test is then performed to determine whether the null hypothesis can be rejected or accepted based on the critical probability (p-value) of 0.05. A calculated probability of less than 0.05 ($p < 0.05$) is considered statistically significant and allows the rejection of the null hypothesis; hence accepting the alternative hypothesis that there is a statistically significant difference/correlation/association between the variables. In the study by Gecaj-Gashi et al. (2010) there was a calculated p-value of 0.011, that is less than 0.05 and hence the null hypothesis that there is no significant difference can be rejected; it can therefore be concluded that there is a significant difference in the incidence in anti-emetic therapy following isoflurane and propofol anaesthesia. The calculation of this probability value will generally be using specific statistical software and the name and version will be included within the paper; it is also possible to do these calculations by hand. However, this is a lengthy and time-consuming process. ODPs therefore need to be able to consider the descriptive and inferential statistics within the paper as these are key to making a judgement of the significance of the study findings upon practice, so it is important to become familiar with these tests.

## Qualitative research

'Qualitative methods explore people's subjective experiences and opinions in order to better understand and give meaning to social phenomena' (Appleton, 2009: 20). Consequently, qualitative research is highly valuable in operating department practice, where we may seek to determine the patient's lived experience of a particular procedure or experience. The data produced from qualitative studies is typically rich and highly relevant to practitioners, especially as ODPs tend not to receive detailed feedback from patients about their experience in the perioperative environment.

### Methods

Qualitative researchers aim to explore experiences and this is generally achieved using one of three main approaches:

- Ethnography is rooted in anthropology and therefore explores behaviour in the context of the setting in which it occurs. This may be particularly valuable for ODPs as it is recognized that the perioperative environment is a unique environment and hence the ODP may used an ethnographic approach, for example, to explore the behaviour of parents accompanying children into the anaesthetic room via observation and interviews.
- Phenomenology explores peoples' perceptions and lived experiences and so the ODP could use this to gain rich data related to the experiences of patients or students in the perioperative environment; for example, to explore patient's experiences of non-scheduled C-section and the care they received.
- Grounded theory develops theory from social research data and hence differs from other methods that use data to verify theories (Glaser and Strauss, 1999). Grounded theory is a commonly used technique for developing the ODPs' understanding of patient experiences and these studies generally use interviews to collect data from people who have undergone a specific procedure or care in a specific environment (e.g. day surgery) and this is then used to develop theories and hypothesis.

### Sampling

Qualitative research is concerned with gaining detailed information about very specific experiences and therefore will collect data from a relatively small sample (generally less than 10) of participants. Consequently, ODPs' conducting qualitative research will need to select participants who are suited to the study aim and therefore studies generally adopt a purposive sampling technique to select participants who can provide the required information.

### Data collection and analysis

The aim of qualitative research is to collect detailed data and hence the ODP researcher will need to select a tool that elicits depth; consequently interviews and focus groups are a common method of data collection for qualitative studies. There are a range of different approaches to interviews; for example, structured and semi-structured interviews, and the researcher will identify the most appropriate for their study. The data is usually collected by tape-recording the participant(s) and this is later transcribed for analysis. It is generally considered beneficial for the researcher to transcribe their own recordings so that they become more familiar with the data and can listen to differences in vocal expression. The analysis of qualitative data is complex and generally involves identifying themes in the data; coding and triangulation may also be used and so it is important to discuss the analysis of data with a supervisor before commencing any qualitative study.

## Mixed-methods research

Mixed-methods research is becoming increasingly recognized as valuable, particularly in healthcare research where we often want to understand the scale of the issue as well as the patient experience and therefore mixed methods utilizes the advantages of both the quantitative and qualitative approaches (Östlund et al., 2011). It may also be argued that the term 'mixed methods' also relates to studies that combine two qualitative or two quantitative methods (within-paradigm research) (Morse, 2010). For example, the ODP may want to research surgical site infection (SSI) and may therefore want to collect data regarding the incidence and severity of SSI (quantitative) and also find out what the patient experience is (this could be collected quantitatively using a survey or qualitatively using interviews for example).

There are a number of definitions of mixed methods and there is often some overlap with a multiple method approach where two research projects are included within the same study; however, it has been recognized that a true mixed-methods approach has a primary philosophical approach with a secondary approach that explores this further (Driessnack et al., 2007; Morse, 2010). A mixed-method design therefore 'consists of a complete method (i.e. the core component), plus one (or more) incomplete method(s) (i.e. the supplementary component[s]) that cannot be published alone, within a single study' (Morse and Niehaus, 2009: 9). Therefore in the ODP example of SSI research, the quantitative method collecting objective data would be the primary approach and the exploration of the patient experience forms the secondary approach.

The validity of this mixed-methods approach to research has been widely debated however it is considered to be a pragmatic approach (Mendlinger and Cwikel, 2008) that is particularly useful in healthcare research because of the complexity of the research questions posed (Östlund et al., 2011). In addition to the complexity of the research questions, funding bodies have also expressed a preference for healthcare research that uses different methods for data collection and considers aspects of both biomedical and social science (Tritter, 2007). There are a number of commonly employed methodological approaches to mixed-methods studies (Tritter, 2007):

- Quantitative + qualitative: This approach starts with a quantitative study that initially collects data; for example, the frequency of a phenomenon or biological/physiological data; the second phase then uses a qualitative approach to explore the experience of the individuals concerned in depth. For example, the ODP may use this approach to explore PONV as the first stage could use a large-scale quantitative approach to collect data about the incidence, severity and treatment of PONV and the second qualitative stage could explore the patient experience and impact upon recovery through an interview approach.
- Qualitative + quantitative: This approach uses an initial qualitative approach to identify key themes that then informs the development of the data collection tool for the larger-scale quantitative component. This could be employed, for example, to determine the student experience of pre-registration ODP education by conducting some initial interviews or focus groups and then using the key themes to produce a questionnaire that would be circulated to a large number of ODP students.
- Qualitative + qualitative (QUAL + qual): This approach uses a standard qualitative method as the primary method (e.g. phenomenology, ethnography, grounded theory), which is supplemented by a component from another method, for example focus groups or observations (Morse, 2010).

The analysis and reporting of results from mixed-methods studies is challenging and it has been shown that a separate analysis of the quantitative and qualitative data is common; in addition, there is often a lack of clarity whether reported results originate from the quantitative or qualitative component (Östlund et al., 2011). It has been suggested that triangulation should be employed to analyse the multiple data sets as this process is believed to produce a stronger conclusion when the results are convergent; however, this will not always be the case and the two methods may report disparate results (Al-Hamdan and Anthony, 2010). When planning a mixed-methods study therefore the ODP should consider the data analysis early in the process and discuss this with their supervisor as this investment early in the project will enhance the work overall.

Mixed-methods research is an evolving approach to perioperative research that can result in valuable information. However, as a developing approach, it presents a number of challenges regarding the combining of two distinctly different paradigms and the resulting data analysis. It is therefore essential that these processes are clearly described within the paper and that the origin of the results are clearly presented (Östlund et al., 2011). Despite these challenges though, mixed-methods research has the potential to make a valuable contribution to the ODP body of knowledge.

## Literature review

Literature reviews are a highly valuable form of research as they effectively collate, summarize and critically discuss key information about the chosen topic. They also form the first stage of a primary research project, as it is necessary to review what is already known about a topic before starting a primary research project. The process of literature review therefore is important to all ODPs both in the development of their own practice and in the advancement of our profession through undertaking literature review for publication in professional journals. Reading published literature reviews is also valuable for ODPs as they provide an analytical review of a chosen topic that allows the reader to get a good understanding of the current research that they can use to inform their own practice.

### Narrative review

Narrative reviews are the most straightforward type of literature review and are similar in format and process to some academic assignments. You will find a number of narrative reviews published in journals and they will provide a broad review about a particular topic. The aim of a narrative review is to illustrate the development of concepts, theories and methods within a specific topic area; the review will therefore synthesize and discuss the previous research and considers it within the current context and within the context in which the original literature was produced to interpret the information (Jones, 2007). The nature of the narrative review however is that it does not follow a strict process to identify and select the articles for inclusion nor do these articles undergo a rigorous appraisal process. For these reasons narrative reviews will be most commonly used by ODPs to update knowledge rather than to inform or change practice.

### Systematic literature review

Systematic literature reviews (SLRs) aim to answer a clearly defined question and are considered to be more reliable than narrative literature reviews due to the explicit methodological rigour that 'limits bias and improves reliability' (Smith and Dixon, 2007: 68), allows the study to be repeatable and demonstrates a scientific approach to the research (The Cochrane Collaboration, 2012). SLRs are therefore a more robust approach to literature reviews and this is important when the findings of the research can be used to inform clinical practice; it is therefore common practice for undergraduate dissertations for ODPs to use the SLR approach.

An SLR should attempt to be as exhaustive as possible to minimize the risk of failing to identify relevant studies (CRD, 2009) and therefore the ODP should search a full range of electronic journal databases, these will be accessible via university e-resources or via an NHS Athens account. In addition to searching electronic journal databases, the ODP will also perform a citation search to identify any potentially relevant papers that have not been identified in the initial searches. While a citation search may identify a number of relevant papers, the nature of the search prevents the identification of recent papers, as they cannot be cited in older publications (CRD, 2009) and therefore this needs to be considered in the context of the study. Google Scholar may also be a useful resource as it includes a range of publication formats including peer-reviewed papers (Bell, 2005) and while it may not be possible to obtain full text for every article, these can generally be ordered via university or hospital libraries.

SLRs generally start with an initial low-precision, high-yield search using key words. However, these searches will result in a considerable number of results, and hence it will then be necessary to narrow this by using a high-precision, low-yield strategy (Smith and Dixon, 2009). It is at this point that Boolean operators (AND, OR, NOT) will be used to combine the terms above to narrow the search; a summary of this process is included in the published article as the methodology. Once a number of studies have been obtained, the papers for inclusion are selected in accordance with strict inclusion and exclusion criteria appropriate to the research question. For example, the ODP may consider it appropriate to include only in-patients, or patients over 18; alternatively, you may exclude emergency cases if the focus of your SLR is elective procedures.

---

**Stop and think**

If you wanted to explore the post-operative recovery after laparotomy as a research project:

- What search terms would you use? How many different words might be relevant to recovery – consider pain? Analgesia (as a requirement for more analgesia would be due to higher pain scores)? PONV? Sickness?
- Who would you include or exclude? Would you want to exclude emergency surgery (what category?) as they may have been less prepared?

There is no absolute right or wrong answer as long as the papers you find are relevant to the research question and that you can justify the inclusion and exclusion criteria.

---

The papers selected for inclusion then undergo a rigorous critical appraisal process to asses validity and reliability. It is considered good practice to have a minimum of two researchers appraising the papers independently and agreeing the results to reduce subjectivity, bias and error (CRD, 2009; Parahoo, 2006). However, this is not possible when conducting an SLR as part of a university programme of study. Following this appraisal the researcher will identify key themes in the literature and critical analysis of these will form the main body of the SLR. This critical analysis will synthesize the data presented in the selected papers and the quality of these studies; identifying relationships between findings and considering the impact of any methodological limitations and identifying areas for further research will be addressed within this discussion. To aid this reporting of SLRs to the Preferred Reporting Items for Systematic Reviews and Meta-Analyses (PRISMA) statement may be beneficial. This is a 27-item checklist that was developed to improve the quality of reporting of systematic reviews and meta-analyses (Moher et al., 2009).

While SLRs utilize existing published literature, they are also subject to critical appraisal and hence may vary in quality due to either the review methodology or the quality of the studies included. Methodical limitations may be also the result of bias introduced by the researcher and hence the ODP must be aware that published SLRs should still be read critically. SLRs typically include only peer-reviewed papers but this results in publication bias within the study, as the only research considered is that which has been published in academic journals. To eliminate publication bias it is necessary to compare published data with unpublished studies (CRD, 2009). However, locating suitable unpublished data can be challenging and such studies may not have been subject to the same quality assurance procedures; for example, ethical approval or peer review. Many SLRs include only articles written in English and this introduces language bias because research with statistically significant results is more likely to be published in English language journals than those that do not have significant results thus resulting in potential bias in the review conclusions (CRD, 2009). However, there are a number of practical considerations if this bias is to be avoided. Best practice for an SLR would therefore include all potentially relevant research, irrespective of language of publication; this however presents a number of practical considerations for the ODP researcher and therefore they should be able to justify the decisions made regarding inclusion and recognize the potential impact upon their work.

SLRs offer the ODP a good opportunity to engage with and undertake a research project without the requirement for ethical approval and hence this is generally a more easily accessible opportunity. Depending on the context of the project, a team can be established and therefore there will be opportunities to work with more experienced researchers to develop skills and confidence in this process, in the same way as discussing your ideas with ODP colleagues who have completed an SLR as part of a dissertation will help to refine your own ideas.

## Critical appraisal of literature

### Purpose

Critical appraisal of literature is a process directly connected to the use of literature review as a research methodology; however, it is also an important skill for ODPs to possess when reading any papers. This is because there is considerable variation in the quality of research studies and any methodological limitation that introduces bias can significantly impact upon the results. A critical assessment of the study quality therefore allows you to determine whether the results can be 'believed' and whether they are sufficient to inform practice (CRD, 2009). In addition, the nature of the online environment means that the majority of ODPs have access to a considerable amount of information and, as you will know, this will vary in quality and accuracy, so it is important that skills of critical appraisal are developed and this process is discussed later in this section.

### Stop and think

When you read journal articles or other material, do you accept it as being correct as it has been published in a peer-reviewed journal? Or do you question the methodology and the validity of the results?

Sometimes people feel that they cannot question these publications as they have achieved publication and are written by individuals who may be more academically qualified. This is not the case however as all ODPs should question the quality of the paper and also consider it in the context of their own practice.

### Principles

The measure of quality is often considered a subjective measure; however, the CRD (2009) have defined some guiding principles when assessing the quality of a research study:

- The suitability of the study design to meet the research objective(s) must be considered, as if the study design is inappropriate then there is little value in continuing with the appraisal.
- Risk of bias must be considered and this may be impacted by a number of methodological considerations, for example blinding or sampling. The general principle regarding bias is that the study must seek to impact the introduction of any variables that could influence the results. For example in a study related to PONV the sample size and sampling strategy would seek to result in two study groups that did not have any demographic differences, as it is known that females have a higher incidence of PONV and therefore if one group had a significantly higher number of female participants this would introduce a bias.
- The selection of outcome measure(s) must be appropriate as this is how the efficacy of the intervention will be measured. In quantitative studies this is particularly important as this is directly connected to sample size when a power analysis is performed.

- The statistical tests performed must be considered in terms of their suitability for the data and study objectives in addition to considering the results obtained. The statistical significance reported should also be considered in the context of the observed differences as there may be a clear observed difference that is not statistically significant and this may suggest an insufficient sample size or that further research is required.
- The quality of the intervention should be considered as there may be anomalies in how the intervention is performed or it may be so different from your own practice area that the results may not be applicable to your own practice.
- The quality of the way the study is reported in the paper must be considered for clarity – is it clear how the study was conducted and what the results are?
- The final consideration is the generalizability of the findings in terms of the wider population and different practice settings. This is also where as an ODP you will consider the applicability to your own practice area and therefore it is important to consider how the context of the research environment may have impacted upon the results.

### Tools

There are a number of tools to guide the critical appraisal process and it is worth spending some time becoming familiar with these to find the ones that you find easiest to use. Some of the commonly used tools are shown below; however, there are a number of additional tools available and hence the inclusion of these should not be considered prescriptive but rather used as a starting point.

- The Critical Appraisal Skills Programme (CASP) tools are frequently used by ODPs as they were designed to support evidence-based practice in healthcare by supporting skill development in the location, appraisal and utilization of evidence in healthcare decision making. There are a number of different CASP checklists for different types of studies (e.g. RCT, systematic reviews and qualitative studies), which can be downloaded from the CASP website (CASP, 2010).
- The LoBiondo-Wood and Haber (2006) guidelines are very detailed and explicitly consider a number of potential threats to the validity of the study. The quantitative tool in particular is particularly suited to the appraisal of papers aiming to test a hypothesis and the ODP may find them particularly useful when appraising laboratory-based studies (e.g. drug research).
- The Litva and Jacoby (2007) tool is designed specifically for the appraisal of qualitative research and therefore the questions are focused upon key aspects of the qualitative methodology (e.g. triangulation).

These tools however are designed for published research/literature review articles. It is also important to apply robust skills of critical appraisal to other publications that do not conform to a standard research paper format. The ODP should also remember that these are purely tools to aid and guide the process and it is possible to appraise a paper critically without using any tool; indeed, as you become more familiar with the process, you will find that reliance on these tools will decrease.

In addition to using research papers, ODPs are used to using clinical guidelines to inform their own practice on a daily basis and these guidelines are also subject to scrutiny and critical appraisal as 'the potential benefits of guidelines are only as good as the quality of the guidelines themselves' (AGREE Research Trust, 2009: 1) and therefore you may want to appraise a guideline either for your own practice or because you are developing a new or similar guideline for your own clinical area. The Appraisal of Guidelines for Research and Evaluation II (AGREE) is an international tool for healthcare practitioners to critique guidelines in addition to aiding the development of guidelines by providing a process for development and a guide for the inclusion and presentation of information (AGREE Research Trust, 2009). These processes are highly relevant to ODPs as skills of critical thinking and appraisal need to be transferable to all areas of practice; understanding the process of guideline development enables you to appreciate how research can be used to inform and enhance patient care on a large scale.

### Stop and think

Why not try reading a journal article using this questioning/critical approach? You may want to download one of the CASP tools to help you or, if not, just consider the research in the context of everything you have read in this chapter. You may prefer to highlight the article or annotate this to identify strengths and limitations.

Having done this, consider – how has reading this article impacted upon your practice? Or do you not consider the article of sufficient quality to affect your practice – does there need to be further research?

Now consider how you can use this process as part of your CPD.

## Clinical audit

Clinical audit is defined as a 'quality improvement process that seeks to improve patient care and outcomes through systematic review of care against explicit criteria and the implementation of change' (National Institute for Health and Clinical Excellence (NICE), 2002: 1). Audit is distinctly different from research; however, the preparation and execution of a clinical audit will employ a number of research principles and skills; hence it has been included within this chapter.

Clinical audit may be undertaken at two levels: national and local. National clinical audits are large-scale projects that can assess compliance with standards on a national level by collecting data submitted by healthcare providers. These national audits aim to influence the development of national standards and processes and hence will still result in an impact at local level (Bullivant and Corbett-Nolan, 2010). A greater number of ODPs however will contribute to local level audits that will measure performance within one hospital or department, or even within one specific operating theatre depending upon the topic.

Audit is a key component of clinical governance as the continuous improvement of services can be directly facilitated via the clinical audit process (Grainger, 2010). Consequently, the importance of clinical audit in governance and service delivery should be recognized by NHS boards as key in monitoring the efficacy of hospital strategy in delivering improvements (Bullivant and Corbett-Nolan, 2010). In addition to these direct improvements, there are a number of additional benefits of audit that can indirectly result in improvements to patient care. For example, it empowers practitioners to assess and adjust their own care, it results in knowledge of the local care delivery and promotes learning (Bowie et al., 2010), all of which can improve the care delivery by both healthcare providers and by individual ODPs.

The explicit relationship between clinical audit and service improvement has resulted in the recognition that audit must be embedded in education to equip ODPs with the confidence and skills to engage with the process (Bowie et al., 2010). The knowledge and skills of clinical audit for ODPs are required at the point of registration (HCPC, 2014) and hence have been embedded in both the Diploma and Degree pre-registration curriculum (College of Operating Department Practitioners (CODP), 2006; CODP, 2011). Despite this however there may be ODPs who feel that they need to update their skills in this area and, while there are a number of different ways of doing this, it is advisable to contact the local hospital audit department as they may offer training sessions or be able to direct ODPs to current audits where they can gain experience of working with a team and then progress to leading an audit. In addition to the need for skill development, there have been a number of additional barriers identified to undertake and implement an audit within the NHS. Research has shown that practitioners report pressure of work and lack of protected time as barriers to engaging in audit (Bowie et al., 2010) and therefore it is important that this is considered at the planning stage and discussed with managers.

**Stop and think**

How often do you think, 'I wonder if we (as a department or profession) are consistently following best practice?'

Or maybe you think that practice is really good, but do you have any evidence to support this?

This could become a topic for clinical audit and if so . . .

How confident would you be in planning and implementing an audit or do you need to develop your knowledge and skills further?

### Differences from research

The primary focus of clinical audit is the improvement of practice, unlike research that seeks primarily to contribute to the body of knowledge. While it may be argued that research may also result in improvements to practice, this is not the fundamental reason for undertaking research.

The audit process is focused on current clinical practice and making observations and comparisons between this and best practice; hence, ethical approval is not required. However, audits should be registered with the local hospital clinical governance department in accordance with any local policy. Although formal ethical approval is not required, there are however a number of ethical and legal issues relating to the audit process; for example, adherence to the Code of Conduct, Performance and Ethics (HCPC, 2012) throughout and ensuring that if patients are asked to comment upon any aspect of the care provided that they are aware that the (anonymized) information may be shared to support service improvement (Patel, 2010).

### Stages and process

Clinical audit follows a set process or cycle that consists of five stages (NICE, 2002), however some texts subdivide these stages further and hence report an increased number of stages in the process.

The first 'preparation' stage of clinical audit is crucial and hence it is important that sufficient time is spent in this stage. Once the purpose of the audit has been clearly identified, the audit team can be established and it is important to consider the skills and expertise required to produce a successful audit; for example, you may require representation from a surgical ward or feel that you need someone with expertise in data analysis. The team can then plan the audit and will need to develop a structure and work plan that includes regular team meetings and while this may be challenging, it is essential to the success of the project.

One of the defining characteristics of clinical audit is the use of explicit criteria and standards against which performance is measured and hence these must be established as the second stage of the process. These criteria are used to assess the quality of care provided and must be explicit statements defining what aspects of perioperative care will be objectively measured (NICE, 2002). These criteria may be derived from a number of sources based on the variable to be measured. For example, local or national guidelines; where no published guidelines exist, the ODP may use evidence-based best practice as the point of reference. The standards define the desired level of success or compliance and are generally expressed as percentages (Ashmore and Ruthven, 2008); for many audits these will often be between 90 per cent and 100 per cent as it would be expected that best practice is consistently being adhered to and that failing to adhere is attributed to exceptional circumstances.

Measuring level of performance is a significant part of the process and requires a significant amount of careful planning, as this is where the tools are developed and used to collect data that is then analysed. Clinical audits may be prospective or retrospective and therefore the ODPs needs to develop the tool appropriately depending on the approach; both approaches have strengths and limitations therefore the team needs to consider that is most suited to the topic and will provide the required data most effectively. The data collection tool is then developed and this is essential to ensure the success of the audit and therefore the tool should ask 'relevant, concise and unambiguous questions' (Grainger, 2010: 32). For some audit topics relating to national guidelines, there are set audit tools available that should be used and hence this should be confirmed prior to starting to develop your own. The data is then collected from the agreed sample of patients, based on a set inclusion or exclusion criteria, throughout the audit period (NICE, 2002); this data is then analysed and the results compared with the criteria and standards.

Audit is a quality improvement process and therefore once the results have been analysed, it is essential that an action plan is developed to make improvements and that this focuses on the areas of practice that have led to the poor audit outcome (Copeland, 2005). The required actions will depend on the audit results; however, these typically involve staff education and training and possible introduction of or revision of systems of practice through changes to local or national policy (Ashmore and Ruthven, 2008). The ODP may therefore deliver additional training or write/update a departmental policy as one of the actions from the audit.

Sustaining improvement is the final stage of the clinical audit process as, having completed the work involved in the audit, it is important that this results in a sustained improvement in practice. While it may be argued that it is the responsibility of individual perioperative practitioners to follow the changes to process, it is also important that this is monitored and hence a follow-up audit after three to six months is usual. In addition to following up with another audit, continued activities to promote awareness and engagement with the changes may be beneficial in the ongoing service improvement.

## Conclusion

This chapter has aimed to review key principles related to research and ODPs and hopefully has contextualized some key concepts. It is sometimes believed that in order to conduct research you need to have completed a doctorate or a Master's degree or that research is only ever conducted as part of a formal academic award; however it is hoped that this chapter has demonstrated that this is not the case and there are a number of ways for ODPs to become engaged with research. Research is rarely undertaken in a solitary manner and, therefore, if you feel that this is an area you want to develop, you may want to see what opportunities there are to engage with projects at your place of work or study as this will help in the development of your knowledge and skills as a researcher.

It is important that ODPs recognize that engagement with research is part of the professional role and that reading research papers is essential to ensure that professional knowledge is current and that the best care is delivered to our patients. As you progress through your ODP career it is important to continue to question practice and address this through literature or maybe undertaking your own research project as it is only through these processes that our practice and our profession will continue to develop.

## Key points

- Engaging with research to deliver evidence-based care is an essential part of the professional role of the ODP.
- Research aims to contribute to the body of knowledge, however, for healthcare practitioners it also aims to improve patient care and service delivery.
- There are two distinctly different overarching philosophical standpoints that have defined the paradigms of research and resulted in the quantitative and qualitative approaches.
- Literature reviews are important for the development of professional knowledge and are frequently conducted to inform and set standards for practice.
- It is essential for ODPs to develop skills of critical appraisal to be able to review information in a critical manner in order to be able to assess whether it is pertinent to their practice setting.
- Clinical audit is a key component of clinical governance and is used to review practice against set standards and make improvements.

## References and further reading

AGREE Research Trust (2009) *Appraisal of Guidelines for Research & Evaluation II*. Available online at http://www.agreetrust.org (accessed 19 May 2013).

Al-Hamdan, Z. and Anthony, D. (2010) 'Deciding on a mixed-methods design in doctoral study', *Nurse Researcher*, 18 (1): 45–56.

Appleton, J.V. (2009) 'Starting a new research project', in Neale, J. (ed.) *Research Methods for Health and Social Care*. Basingstoke: Palgrave Macmillan.

Ashmore, S. and Ruthven, T. (2008) 'Clinical audit: a guide', *Nursing Management*, 15 (1): 18–22.

Bell, J. (2005) *Doing Your Research Project* (4th edn). Maidenhead: Open University Press.

Beyea, S.C. (2004) 'Evidence-based practice in perioperative nursing', *American Journal of Infection Control*, 32: 97–100.

Bowie, P., Bradley, N.A. and Rushmer, R. (2010) 'Clinical audit and quality improvement – time for a rethink?', *Journal of Evolution in Clinical Practice*, 18: 42–48.

Broom, A. and Willis, E. (2007) 'Competing paradigms in health research', in Saks, M. and Allsop, J. (eds) *Researching Health; Qualitative, Quantitative and Mixed Methods*. London: Sage Publications.

Bullivant, J. and Corbett-Nolan, A. (2010) *Clinical Audit: A Simple Guide for NHS Boards & Partners*. London: Good Governance Institute and Healthcare Quality Improvement Partnership. Available online at http://www.hqip.org.uk/assets/Guidance/HQIP-Clinical-Audit-Simple-Guide-online1.pdf (accessed 14 May 2013).

Centre for Reviews and Dissemination (CRD) (2009) *Systematic Reviews: CRD's Guidance for Undertaking Reviews in Health Care*. York: CRD. Available online at http://www.york.ac.uk/inst/crd/pdf/Systematic_Reviews.pdf (accessed 14 May 2013).

College of Operating Department Practitioners (CODP) (2006) *The Diploma in Higher Education in Operating Department Practice Curriculum Document*. London: CODP.

College of Operating Department Practitioners (CODP) (2011) *Bachelor of Science (Hons) in Operating Department Practice – England, Northern Ireland and Wales; Bachelor of Science in Operating Department Practice – Scotland*. London: CODP.

Copeland, G. (2005) *A Practical Handbook for Clinical Audit, Clinical Governance Support Team*. Available online at http://www.hqip.org.uk/assets/Downloads/Practical-Clinical-Audit-Handbook-CGSupport.pdf (accessed 14 May 2013).

Courtney, M., Rickard, C., Vickerstaff, J. and Court, A. (2010) 'Evidence-based nursing practice', in Courney M. and McCutcheon H. (eds) *Using Evidence to Guide Nursing Practice*. Sydney: Churchill Livingstone.

Critical Appraisal Programme (CASP) (2010) *Critical Appraisal Skills Programme: Making Sense of Evidence*. Available online at http://www.casp-uk.net (accessed 14 May 2013).

Department of Health (DH) (2005) *Research Governance Framework for Health and Social Care* (2nd edn). London: DH.

Driessnack, M., Sousa, V.D. and Mendes, I.A.A. (2007) 'An overview of research designs relevant to nursing. Part 3: mixed and multiple methods', *Revista Latino-Americana de Enfermagem*, 15 (5): 1046–49.

Galser, B.G. and Strauss, A.L. (1999) *Discovery of Grounded Theory: Strategies for Qualitative Research*. Chicago, IL: AldineTransaction.

Gecaj-Gashi, A., Hashimi, M., Baftiu, N., Salihu, S., Terziqi, H. and Bruqi, B. (2010) 'Propofol vs isoflurane anesthesia-incidence of PONV in patients at maxillofacial surgery', *Advances in Medical Science*, 55 (2): 308–12.

Glasziou, P., Del Mar, C. and Salisbury, J. (2003) *Evidence-based Medicine Workbook: Finding and Applying the Best Research Evidence to Improve Patient Care*. London: BMJ Publishing Group.

Grainger, A. (2010) 'Clinical audit: shining a light on good practice', *Nursing Management*, 17 (4): 30–33.

Health and Care Professional Council (HCPC) (2012) *Standards of Conduct, Performance and Ethics*. London: HCPC.

Health and Care Professional Council (HCPC) (2014) *Standards of Proficiency; Operating Department Practitioners*. London: HCPC.

Health Research Authority (2013) *National Research Ethics Service*. Available online at http://www.nres.nhs.uk (accessed 14 May 2013).

Jones, K. (2007) 'Doing a literature review in health', in Saks, M. and Allsop, J. (eds) *Researching Health, Qualitative, Quantitative and Mixed Methods*. London: Sage Publications.

Katz, M.H. (2006) *Study Design and Statistical Analysis: A Practical Guide for Clinicians*. Cambridge: Cambridge University Press.

Länsimies-Antikainen, H., Laitinen, T., Rauramaa, R. and Pietilä, A-M. (2009) 'Evaluation of informed consent in health research: a questionnaire survey', *Scandinavian Journal of Caring Studies*, 24: 56–64.

Litva, A. and Jacoby, A. (2007) 'Qualitative research: critical appraisal', in Craig J.V. and Smyth R.L. (eds) *The Evidence-based Practice Manual for Nurses* (2nd edn). Edinburgh: Churchill Livingstone.

LoBiondo-Wood, G. and Haber, J. (2006) *Nursing Research Methods and Critical Appraisal for Evidence-based Practice*. St. Louis, MO: Mosby Elsevier.

Mendlinger, S. and Cwikel, J. (2008) 'Spirallying between qualitative and quantative data on women's health behaviours: a double helix model for mixed methods', *Qualitative Health Reserach*, 18 (2): 280–93.

Moher, D., Liberati, A., Tetzlaff, J. and Altman, D.G. (2009) 'Preferred reporting items for systematic reviews and meta-analyses: the PRISMA statement', *British Medical Journal*, 339: 332–36.

Morse, J. (2010) 'Simultaneous and sequential qualitative mixed method designs', *Qualitative Enquiry*, 16 (6): 483–91.

Morse, J.M. and Niehaus, L. (2009) *Principles and Procedures of Mixed Methods Design*. Walnut Creek, CA: Left Coast Press.

National Institute for Health and Clinical Excellence (NICE) (2002) *Principles for Best Practice in Clinical Audit*. Oxford: Radcliffe Medical Press.

Östlund U., Kidd L., Wengström, Y. and Rowa-Dewar, N. (2011) 'Combining qualitative and quantitative research within mixed method research design: a methodological review', *International Journal of Nursing Studies*, 48: 369–83.

Parahoo, K. (2006) *Nursing Research; Principles, Process and Issues* (2nd edn). Basingstoke: Palgrave Macmillan.

Patel, S. (2010) 'Achieving quality assurance through clinical audit', *Nursing Management*, 17 (3): 28–35.

Prasun, M.A. (2013) 'Evidence-based practice', *Heart & Lung*, 42: 84.

Sackett, D.L., Straus, S.E., Richardson, W.S., Rosenberg, W. and Hayes, R.B. (2001) *Evidence Based Medicine: How to Practice and Teach EBM*. London: Churchill Livingstone.

Smith, L. and Dixon, L. (2009) 'Systematic reviews', in Neale, J. (ed.) *Research Methods for Health and Social Care*. Basingstoke: Palgrave-Macmillan.

Strange, F. (2001) 'The persistence of ritual in nursing practice', *Clinical Effectiveness in Nursing*, 5 (4): 177–83.

The Cochrane Collaboration (2012) *Cochrane Reviews* [online]. Available at http://www.cochrane.org/cochrane-reviews (accessed 24 June 2012).

Tritter, J. (2007) 'Mixed methods and multidisciplinary research in health care', in Saks, M. and Allsop, J. (eds) *Researching Health: Qualitative, Quantitative and Mixed Methods*. London: Sage Publications.

# 4 Patient safety and the Operating Department Practitioner

## Keith Underwood

---

**Key topics**

- The World Health Organization (WHO) Safe Surgery Checklist

- Human factors

  ○ The human element
  ○ The power gradient, personalities and staff interaction
  ○ Devices and button pressing

  ○ Drug administration and Tall Man lettering

- Root cause analysis (RCA)

- Safeguarding issues

  ○ Vulnerable adults
  ○ Children
  ○ Learning disabilities

---

## Introduction

In this chapter we examine several different aspects relating to patient safety. Although they are all individual subjects in their own right, and they build into one subject, there is no stand-alone subject that encompasses patient safety as an entirety. So, to make sure we have the correct knowledge base when dealing with patients, we must not only understand some of the basic principles around the subjects covered, but should also recognize that this is not an exhaustive list of patient safety issues.

## Why is this relevant?

Patient safety has always been a big issue, but in the modern operating department the overall subject of patient safety is a key issue for Operating Department Practitioners (ODPs). The first thing to remember is that patient safety in the operating theatre is not a management issue; it is an individual practitioner issue irrespective of grade or title. For the multidisciplinary team members to work effectively and to provide the best care for the patient, we must understand issues around patient safety and communication skills. Without these the team becomes a group of individuals working in the same room, but would they be working effectively and to the same common goals?

## The WHO Safe Surgery Checklist

One of the main patient safety initiatives to be introduced into the modern operating theatre is the WHO Safe Surgery Saves Lives campaign. Within individual clinical areas through the country, it will probably have been introduced at different levels and with different emphasis within the process. Most probably for the majority of areas, using the patient checklist section would have been the main emphasis as the use of a 19-item checklist has been shown to reduce complications and mortality associated with surgery by over 30 per cent. When looking at the process of introducing the WHO documentation Lamb-Richardson and Underwood (2010) believe that for the project to be successful, it is essential to have staff acceptance of the process and documentation. But for the system to work in its entirety all three phases of the process should be introduced and used effectively with the multi-disciplinary team and therefore the ODP needs to engage fully with this process in each of the phases. These three phases are: the *team brief* (prior to the start of the list); the *patient checklist* (during the patient episode); and the *debrief* (to be completed at the end of the list). We look at some of these aspects later as they link into other discussion notes.

- *Team brief* – ideally this should be completed with all members of the team present prior to sending for the first patient. During the team brief, issues should be raised in relation to equipment availability, patient position on the list, for example, should the patient be first or last due to latex allergies or MRSA status, issues relating to available time and/or availability of specialist staff needed and potential complications. Discussing all these considerations should make the list or individual case run more smoothly.
- *Patient checklist* – the checklist is a 19-item list that should be completed for all patients entering the operating theatre. This has been designed so that all members of the team are not only aware of which patient is going to undergo what procedure, but also so that all team members are aware of who the other team members are. For the majority of the time this is probably a given, but the ODP needs to think about when specialists or unknown individuals arrive within their list. Do we know just who they are; are they students, specialists, visitors or company representatives for example?

    The checklist is split into three defined sections: before induction of anaesthesia; before skin incision; and before the patient leaves the operating room. To optimize patient safety, all three sections should be completed at the appropriate time within the patient episode. For complete- ness it should also be remembered that appropriate documentation should be completed prior to the patient leaving the post-anaethesia care unit (PACU) (recovery) and form part of the hand- over to the ward staff.
- *Debrief* – this should be completed at the end of the 'list' to discuss any issues that arose during it; for example, list optimization, caseload, availability of specialist equipment and/or staff, or crit- ical incidents. It is hoped that for the majority of the time there will be very little to discuss if anything at all, but the opportunity should be made available for any of the team to discuss any issue irrespective of how trivial others might find it. After all, the purpose of the debrief is to look at making the best use of resources so enhancing the smooth running of the list.

If an incident of any type is to be discussed and/or reviewed, then the use of an appropriate RCA tool might well help. Obviously this will depend on the incident and the severity of the outcome or poten- tial outcome. The use of an appropriate RCA tool is discussed later in this chapter.

There will be certain acute circumstances where it becomes impractical to complete the WHO document in the way it was designed. In these circumstances it should be looked upon as a tool to be used as well as possible. The WHO has acknowledged this and as part of their information package also discusses the emergency patient.

### Stop and think

Think of the modern operating theatre as a Formula 1 pit stop. The driver and car is the patient, and the pit crew are the theatre staff. Each member of the pit crew knows exactly what to do when the F1 driver turns up. They all have their own individual roles, but work and communicate as a team to get the car out of the pits in the quickest possible time, without incident, and working as safely as possible. Now we are not saying that we should get our patient through the department in an equivalent time of, say, three to four seconds, but the principles of teamwork and communication are exactly the same. We should remember that communication could be verbal and non-verbal, and dependent on the situation one will be used more than the other.

Think about when you have been working in one of the ODP roles, for example you may be scrubbed; do you know what the other members of the team are trying to achieve? How effectively does the team communicate so that you can all perform your individual roles while working towards the common goal of the team?

## Human factors

Human factors' origin is in the design and use of aircraft during the Second World War to improve aviation safety. Since then the term 'human factors' has been expanded to incorporate not only design features but also non-technical skills training and crew resource management, and has been expanded from the aviation industry, both civilian and military, to engineering, motor sport, overseas disaster, management, the nuclear power industry, the list goes on. More recently, medicine has picked up on the term and it is now used internationally. As stated previously, human factors as a concept has many associated arms so, for the purpose of this section, we concentrate on just a couple of them. The main emphasis is on crew resource management and teamwork and communication skills, and we also explore, in part, equipment design and use.

The Clinical Human Factors Group, cited by The Empowered Patient Coalition (2013) states that:

Human factors are all the things that make us different from logical, completely predictable machines. How we think and relate to other people, equipment and our environment. It is about how we perform in our roles and how we can optimize that performance to improve safety and efficiency. In simple terms it's the things that affect our personal performance.

There is a generalized thought in the aviation industry that there are defined issues relating to human factors, these are commonly known as the 'dirty dozen', and link very well into human factors within medicine. These so-called dirty dozen are: fatigue; stress; complacency; lack of communication; lack of awareness; distraction; lack of knowledge; lack of teamwork; lack of resources; pressure; lack of assertiveness; and what they call 'norms' (Aviation Knowledge, 2010). From looking at the aviation's dirty dozen you could place all of these factors into the modern operating theatre and probably into most if not all other clinical areas of work within the modern hospital environment.

While working within a team we should be aware of four defining factors. These are: *situational awareness* – do all staff understand just what is happening at any particular time?; *decision making;* – are the right people making the right decision at the right time?; *communication and teamwork* – do individual team members communicate appropriately, and are they working as a team?, and *leadership* – just who is the leader, and are they the leader all of the time? (Flin et al., 2008).

Looking initially at the first in the list, situational awareness, a BBC2 *Horizon* programme shown on the 13 March 2012, entitled 'Out of control?', showed that the majority of the time it is our unconscious mind that takes in more than our conscious mind, stating that the conscious mind can only deal with two or three different things at any one time. So, it is important that as a member of the multidisciplinary team, we communicate effectively on any issues that might arise, remembering that just because we saw what was going on does not necessarily mean that others did as well. The other thing to remember about the subconscious part of the brain is that occasionally it will come up with the 'a-ha' moment where it sees something that it wants you to respond to. It might not click straight away just what it is, but it has done it for a reason, so look out for it.

- Decision making either within the team or as an individual can be hampered because of many reasons. Although not an exhaustive list these could include: not enough information available at the time; not sure if you are the right person to make the decision; inexperience in the situation; and unsure of the team dynamics and individuals' abilities.
- Communication and teamwork has always been there within the operating theatre team, to a greater or lesser degree dependent on the area, and it would be impossible to run a theatre list without it. How well this works will depend on the team and the individual personalities within that team. This is explored later in the chapter.
- Leadership within the team can be a controversial matter. Who is the team leader and is there more than one team leader at any one time? Is there more than one team in the operating theatre; for example, the surgical team and the anaesthetic team? How often does the team leader role move from one person to another? Is it always the 'senior' staff member leading the team? Again, this is explored in more detail later.

### Stop and think

We should remember that we have known about 'human factors' for a lot longer than the term has been used. This is quite evident because of how simple things that we use every day have developed. For instance, we have all in the past used a pencil either to draw or to write with. Have we got things wrong when doing this? Well, yes, we have. So what did we do about it? Well, we put a rubber on the end of the pencil, so assisting with fixing an error we might have done. Did the pencil do the error, or was it the individual using the pencil? Well, it was the individual, so this is a human error. Why do you think that bumpers have been placed on cars, buses, trucks, and so on? It is because the human interaction/human factor of the device; namely, the driver, is more than likely to be the instigator of the incident than the device itself. This is also why we have safety catches on weapons. Items like this are just taken for granted in a lot of the things we see and use in the modern world.

Thinking about these examples where human factors have been identified and solutions instigated, what healthcare examples can you think of, and how have you modified your own practice to reduce risk?

### The power gradient, personalities and staff interaction

Personalities within any team, but especially a multidisciplinary team, play a big part in any communication barriers. Within the theatre team, you could have senior and experienced medical, nursing and ODP staff who have significant competence and the confidence to say how they feel about any given situation. This might also be a team that is used to working together and understands each other's idiosyncrasies; by virtue of this, this team will probably work well in both the routine and stressful situations. It is not uncommon for staff that work closely together and have clinical experience to be able to anticipate each other's needs. The anaesthetic practitioner who goes and gets the atropine just before the anaesthetist asks for it, and the scrub practitioner who places the correct instrument into the surgeon's hand without any verbal indication as to what they require, are all signs of experience and teamwork. But then there is the other side of the coin. These could be experienced individuals who have not worked together within this team, or one inexperienced individual who is working within a recognized team. Either way, the team dynamics and communication for these will be different from the closely knit team. This is just being human. On the whole, we like to work with people we know and like, but especially in a stressful situation where we might be looking for guidance/leadership and/or where we take the lead role.

Situational awareness is an issue with all staff within the multidisciplinary team irrespective of grade or profession, so what one person sees another might potentially miss. It may be suggested that if we analysed critical incidents where, for example, wrong site surgery occurred, it could be found on occasions that an individual within the team had spotted the mistake but did not say anything. The reasons for such omissions are varied, but would probably include the individual not wanting to speak up because of inexperience, and where they feel they sit on the 'power gradient' within the team. We are all probably aware of the commonly used phrase: '*We are all equal, but some are more equal than others.*' However, to flatten this 'power gradient' we all need to realize that the phrase should be: '*We are all equal in a given situation.*' The 'power gradient' within an operating theatre is as old as the operating theatre itself; there is a perceived ladder of rank of professionals who work together in the perioperative environment, and different roles may be perceived to be at different levels within this rank. However, for a team to work more effectively this 'power gradient' needs to be flattened. Within any team when managing a critical situation, there needs to be a leader who the team looks to for instruction. Within the operating theatre there might even be two at any one time such as the anaesthetist and the surgeon. But what we need to remember is that no individual can see and/or hear everything when concentrating on completing complex practical tasks within a stressful situation and so it is therefore of paramount importance that all members of the team are empowered to say what they think, and when they think it should be said. This is flattening the power gradient. Anecdotal evidence from consultant surgeons and anaesthetists suggests that medical staff expect other team members to vocalize their concerns irrespective of grade; with some medical staff considering it negligent if the team member did not raise concerns at the time of the incident.

### Stop and think

When looking at how well teams work together and team dynamics, there will always be a difference between an acute and a routine situation. Why?

One thing to consider when the multidisciplinary team with different levels of experience are working together is why individuals might not air their individual thoughts. So consider this, if you are walking through the London Underground on your way to a platform, and say you are not used to visiting London, you know the platform is in a particular direction, but you are unsure exactly which turns to take and when, then you will tend to go with the flow of the other commuters even if the way they are going indicates that it is a 'no entry'. You could well be doing this, as you believe that others must be right and know a short cut because they are 'more experienced'. So, a question for you to think about; could this work the same in a clinical situation where a less confident member of the team is swayed into a decision because others with 'more experience' have come up with that particular decision? Potentially, this could be a form of quorum threshold, where you make your decision based on what others have decided and not on what you think. This has undoubtedly happened in the past within a clinical emergency situation.

### Devices and button pressing

The issue of human factors also falls into the design and use of medical devices, as with aircraft manufacture. Button configuration on devices can make a difference to how they are used. The ODP will probably find that the modern medical devices for drug and fluid administration; that is, syringe drivers and volumetric infusion pumps, when produced from the same company have a similar if not identical button configuration and screen layout. By doing this, it not only helps with the training requirements for the new device, but can also help when looking at critical incidents. One of the changes you might find in new devices is that the numerical format for programming information has been replaced with up and down arrows/chevrons, a dial-up system or equivalent. This change in inputting required dose and/or volume is because of how we interpret what we do. By using a number pad, there is a higher potential for the wrong amount to be entered, as individuals tend to pay more attention to what they are pressing than to what is on the screen. By using an arrow or chevron or dial-up system, you tend to concentrate more on the display, as your fingers do not tend to move around the keypad quite as much.

Other aspects of future design, especially with syringe drivers and volumetric infusers is associated with logging what has been done and when. Currently, most new devices have a memory that can include: date and time settings for alterations in rate; date and time settings for when an alarm went off, and they also tend to record dose; drug name (we look more closely at drug names later); and bolus time and amount. One thing that is missing from most if not all of this particular type of device is that it does not record who the operator was and hence it may be that future volumetric and syringe drivers will have the capability to record which individual staff member made the alterations to the device. This could be achieved by using staff ID cards as the source to log on and off to such devices, especially if an employing organization uses a barcode system that can be transferred to staff identification. There may also be developments in fingerprint recognition that would assist with the device log in process. By using either of these formats, there is also the possibility that individuals could be locked out of an individual or a group of devices if they have not had an appropriate initial and/or update/refresher training session or revalidated competence. This system is available now for some devices and where there is an appropriate Wi-Fi and e-Learning system available within the organization. For this to be developed further, however, technology in medical devices needs to catch up with smart phone and tablet technology.

### Tall Man lettering

While looking at the human factors aspect, there is also a potential problem (Underwood, 2012) with misreading drug information. According to the Medical Protection Society (MPS) (2012), The National Patient Safety Agency (NPSA), which was abolished on 1 June 2012, had operated a National Reporting and Learning Service (NRLS) that received about 5,000 reports a month about patient safety incidents related to medication.

'Tall Man lettering' was introduced into the pharmaceutical industry some time ago to differentiate between 'look alike' and 'sound alike' drug names, and was advocated by the then National Patient Safety Agency. You will find Tall Man lettering is becoming more frequently used within the pharmaceutical industry, and it is also being incorporated not only in both syringe drivers and volumetric infusion devices as part of their device drug libraries, but also on the electronic pharmacy lists for wards and departments, and also on the labelling of the drug boxes themselves. As an example, as part of a recent procurement of the CareFusion Alaris GH+ syringe driver, 30 pre-programmed drug names were added to the device. Some of the drugs protocols pre-programmed are: AMINOphylline; AMIODARone; DOBUTamine; DOPamine; doPEXamine; FUROSemide; and NORadrenaline. This short list shows how they are shown on the devices using Tall Man lettering. So, if you see drug names with an unusual typeface setting, it might not be a misprint, it might be Tall Man lettering and is there to help you correctly identify the drug of choice, so making drug administration safer for the patient. You might also see the use of different colours for the text on the drug packaging. This is also part of the Tall Man system.

**Stop and think**

Have you come across Tall Man lettering within your work place? If so, do others you work with understand its use?

# RCA

There are numerous sources of information regarding RCA and so the key point to remember is that it is not important which system is used, but what is important is how well it is used; you will get better results using a simple system well, than you would by using a complex system badly. Within the system we look at later, there are six key factors that will need to be considered. These are: measurements; materials; personnel; environment methods; and machines. By using a process as simple as a Fishbone/Ishikawa diagram it is relatively easy to start an RCA.

Adverse incident, significant event, serious untoward incident, serious incident and the near miss are common terms used generally within an event review analysis. One other that is now used within the National Health Service (NHS) is the 'never event' (Department of Health (DH), 2012). The 'never events' document describes events that should never happen within the NHS as they are considered unacceptable and eminently preventable. Within the 2012/13 edition, there are descriptors for 25 such events, quite a few of which are or could be theatre related and therefore ODPs need to be aware of these.

Two of the key NHS specific definitions are shown in Box 4.1 to help give you a better understanding of the terminology

**Box 4.1 Definitions of common terms used in event review analysis**

| | |
|---|---|
| **Serious Events** | A situation in which one or more patients, or staff are involved in an event that would present a significant danger to patients, visitors or staff, or is likely to generate significant legal, media or other interest which, if not properly managed, may result in loss of the Trust's reputation, services or assets |
| **Near Miss** | An unplanned event that had the potential to cause damage, injury or illness, but on this particular occasion did not |

**Stop and think**

A 'near miss' in aviation terms is defined where planes are within three nautical miles of each other horizontally, or 1,000 feet vertically. So should we have a quantifiable definition of a near miss in the operating theatre? Can you identify a near miss situation relevant to the role of the ODP?

We should also consider the seriousness of the incident, remembering that in any incident it may not include 'damage' to a patient or staff member. The seriousness could be defined as seen in Box 4.2.

**Box 4.2 Categories used to classify the seriousness of an incident**

| | |
|---|---|
| **Major** | This could include penetrating injury, loss of life, causing unconsciousness, loss of sight, additional and/or prolonged treatment |
| **Moderate** | This could include drug administration errors with no lasting effects, verbal or physical abuse or fraud |
| **Minor** | This could include minor theft, slips, trips and falls with little injury or vandalism |

*Note:* These lists are for illustrative purposes only and are not exhaustive.

RCA is a process for looking at all aspects associated with a given situation, analysing any potential and/or actual problems or incidents and developing a plan to ensure wherever practicable that it will not happen again. These situations could be related to a critical incident, serious event, near miss or a recognized never event.

RCA as a process can be conducted at a departmental, Trust, regional, national and even international level. To put this into perspective, an international RCA was completed some years ago and the results have significantly altered the way we all work within the operating department. The outcome of this RCA was the WHO Safe Surgery Initiative.

The overall process of conducting an RCA is not new to healthcare management or the operating theatre. In the past we looked at issues/situations that had occurred, discussed problems and came up with a plan to ensure it did not happen again. With progression, this has now led to a process that needs to be accurately reviewed and documented and where needed reported appropriately be that Trust, regional or potentially nationally. Part of the process is to develop an appropriate action plan that would probably need to be linked to the Trust's risk and legal department. This overall process will probably start with an online reporting system such as the Datix AIRS approach. Which system you use within your clinical area is not important, but what is, is that it is used appropriately and correctly.

If we now consider the six factors mentioned previously and expand them into general operating department terminology, we can see how this RCA framework can work for ODPs and provide information for 'the incident'. An example of this can be seen in Box 4.3.

**Box 4.3 Example of how the RCA framework can be applied to the perioperative environment**

| | |
|---|---|
| **Measurements** | Calibration of instrumentation and/or device, dosage (e.g. mg, mcg, ml, mm), printout from devices, information stored on device |
| **Materials** | Cleaning agents, suppliers, latex in product, control of substances hazardous to health (COSHH) data sheets availability |
| **Personnel** | We may need to consider issues around the time of day (e.g. shift patterns, staffing numbers, appropriate training, skill mix as well as who was there, were there students/learners present and the availability of senior staff) |
| **Environment** | Time of day, temperature, humidity, lighting, just where did the incident occur? |
| **Methods** | Policies local and national, procedures, standard operating procedures, national standards and/or requirements |
| **Machines** | Considers the devices used, servicing records, appropriate training, correct devices for purpose, up-to-date software, device protocols signed off appropriately, completed checklists, brackets/attachments |

There are two points to remember;

1 It is not an exhaustive list for any of the headings; it is intended to develop your thought processes.
2 Depending on the incident not all of the headings will have items to be added. Do not try and find something for each heading, if it is there then that is OK; if it is not, then that is fine too.

To illustrate this further using the RCA process, it can be useful to explore a particular example of an incident that did not result in a long-lasting injury to a patient. While sliding Mr D (anaesthetized), from the bed to the operating table he fell between the two and landed on the floor. So what are the things we need to look at and consider? By using the six factors it will hopefully give us all the information we require.

- Measurement – there is probably nothing within this section of relevance to this case.
- Materials – again, there is nothing of relevance for this section.
- Personnel – for this we would look at the staff involved, their individual experiences, their training requirements and their training status (are they up to date?). Remember that training requirements and training status are very different. For the training we would be looking at current competence around moving and handling and medical devices for all staff that were involved irrespective of grade or profession. We could also consider the time of day as this could have two influencing factors: (1) the amount of available staff; and (2) natural fatigue due to shift patterns.
- Environment – for this we should consider where this occurred, was it a suitable area to perform the move, and the time of day.
- Method – this is probably the most important issue to look at along with the individuals' training. We would be considering if there were any standard operating procedures for the task in hand; that is, moving the patient, what the standard operating procedure states, and if there was evidence of the individuals being aware of them. It is not uncommon for the standard operating procedures to be placed in a departmental folder with a read and sign sheet. If this was the case, then these signature sheets would need to be examined and would be used as part of the overall evidence.
- Machines – again, for this section we would be looking at the training requirements around any medical devices used, and also seeing if there were any faults with the wheel-locking mechanism on the bed or table. This would give us some idea as to whether the two items could be locked in place prior to patient movement. It would be imperative that the devices asset numbers or serial numbers were recorded on any incident form and/or notes so that the appropriate tests could be made as part of the RCA.

We should also be aware that each member of staff involved could well be required to complete a report on the incident that detailed what they did and said prior to and at the time of the incident, in order to gain a full picture.

**Stop and think**

What do you think the probable outcome of the RCA investigation will show for this incident? Will it be a defect in the locking system of the bed and/or table, or will it be a human factors issue?

Looking at individual case studies is a good way of getting a better understanding of the root cause analyses process. To this end, we list below two case studies for you to examine. The first has been completed as an example of the process, whereas the second will give you the opportunity to complete the process on an individual basis. Some prompts have been added to assist in the process.

## Case study 1

History – a 26-year-old female is admitted for a routine minor gynaecological procedure at 07:45 for a list starting at 09:00. There are five cases in total three major surgical procedures and two minor surgical procedures. The team works together on a regular basis and has two students/learners working with them. One is a student ODP; the other is a new healthcare assistant (HCA) to the department. Our patient (Miss X) arrives in the department at 12:15 being last on the list and enters the theatre having been anaesthetized in the anaesthetic room. The WHO documentation is complete and staff are informed that Miss X has an allergy to penicillin and some 'sticky tape'. The student ODP is scrubbed with the registered practitioner supervising her (but not scrubbed). The procedure is almost complete when the theatre co-ordinator comes into the theatre and discusses an emergency that needs to follow this case. The registered practitioner is discussing the pending emergency, so the HCA and the student ODP complete the final count; all is well and the appropriate documentation is completed. The patient recovers with no complications and is then sent to the ward. The emergency is complete and all is well. Four hours after Miss X has returned to the ward, the junior doctor (F2) is called to assess her as she is in pain and is still bleeding per vagina (PV), but not excessively.

*Outcome – a swab was removed by the F2 on PV examination on the ward.*

### Box 4.4 RCA for case study 1

|  | Relevant information |
| --- | --- |
| **Measurements** | Probably nothing for this section |
| **Material** | Probably nothing for this section |
| **Personnel** | The multidisciplinary team including students and learners as part of the team. Had appropriate training been given to all staff? Was there appropriate supervision of staff at all times? Was there any distraction from others while supervising learners? |
| **Environment** | Probably nothing for this section, but consideration might be taken as to the emergency case that needed to be completed. Did they do one case at a time? |
| **Method** | Are all policies and procedures adhered to correctly? Consider the swab and instrument counts, supervision of student and learners, the WHO documentation. |
| **Machines** | Probably nothing for this section |

The main facts for this case study are as follows:

- Was there inappropriate supervision of the learners?
- Should a new HCA be conducting a swab and instrument count with a student ODP?
- Was the WHO documentation completed correctly at the end?
- Was there too much of a distraction while discussing the pending emergency, and was this appropriate at the time?
- Was there enough focus on Miss X by the team?

Prevention of occurrence – being more vigilant when supervising learners and using procedures, process standard operating procedures and documentation appropriately and correctly.

Use the same principles as used in case study 1. So think about the process, what relevant information has been given, but more importantly the information that is not relevant.

## Case study 2

History – a 26-year-old male, Mr Q, is brought into the emergency department after being involved in a road traffic accident (RTA). He is conscious with multiple fractures, one of which is open. The ODP is part of the trauma team who attends accompanied by a student ODP. After initial physical and radiological assessment, it is decided to transfer him 120 miles to a trauma centre with more specialist facilities more suited to Mr Q's needs. All appropriate measures are taken to manage the airway, as ventilation is required for the transfer. Fractures and external bleeding are sorted appropriately for the transfer, and information recorded. Information is passed on to the receiving hospital and appropriate consultant staff. The ambulance is called as a priority 1 call, so arrives at the department within six minutes. Information is given to the paramedic crew, and Mr Q is prepared for transfer and loaded onto the ambulance. Approximately 25 minutes into the journey the ODP notices that the saturations are dropping and then the ventilator alarm sounds indicating low oxygen pressure. It is noted that the oxygen cylinder is empty, so is changed over. During this process a self-inflating bag is used to ventilate Mr Q. Cylinder changed, ventilator reconnected, saturations increase to 100 per cent, all is well. The rest of the journey is uneventful. Handover is completed at the receiving hospital and a decision is made to complete an incident form for the oxygen cylinder.

*Outcome – Mr Q's condition on arrival was unchanged from when they departed the referring hospital; however, the incident on the transfer could have been avoided. Mr Q returned to the referring hospital for recuperation after three surgical procedures. He eventually walked out of hospital and thanked all staff.*

### Box 4.5 RCA for cast study 2

|  | Relevant information (well some, you add the rest) |
| --- | --- |
| **Measurements** | Is there anything relevant for this situation? |
| **Material** | Appropriate availability of oxygen? |
| **Personnel** | Could the time of day have had any influence? |
| **Environment** | Is this a known environment for the ODP and the anaesthetist? Do they understand availability of resources within the ambulance? Had they had appropriate transfer training? |
| **Method** | Transfer protocols used/adhered to? |
| **Machines** | Appropriate training for all involved? |

This case study has been made purposely ambiguous in parts, this is to help you think about the complexity of RCA. Is there a definitive outcome? One thing to remember with this scenario is if you do not come up with a definitive outcome it is not a reflection on your ability, as individuals need to get used to any RCA process. It should also be remembered that RCA should not be conducted in isolation; it is a team, probably a multidisciplinary team process, depending on the situation.

## Safeguarding issues

Safeguarding vulnerable individuals within a healthcare setting falls within the remit of all staff be they clinical or non-clinical. As an overall subject, it is rather like human factors in that there are many subsections. So, for the purposes of this section we look at just three key areas: vulnerable adults, vulnerable children and learning disabilities.

### Vulnerable adults and children

It is important that we have an understanding of some of the basic terminology used (e.g. vulnerable adult, abuse and abuser). Each organization will have a definition they use for each, and although the meanings will be the same, wording will vary slightly through the country, so it is important that you know your own organization's definitions. Examples of the common terminology can be seen in Box 4.6.

**Box 4.6 Common terminology relating to vulnerable adults and children**

| Term | Meaning |
| --- | --- |
| **Vulnerable adult** | An individual who will be over the age of 18 and unable for some reason to look after themselves. This might be because of physical or mental health problems, age, illness or learning disabilities |
| **Abuse** | Where one or more people say or do something that causes physical, mental, emotional or sexual harm to an individual. It can also be where an individual's civil or human rights are violated |
| **Abuser** | Any individual can be an abuser, be they friend, relative, carer or unknown |

### Adult-specific training

Training within organizations would most probably be broken down into set levels for individual staff/practitioner grades. The Association of Directors of Social Services (2005: 20) *Safeguarding Adults: A National Framework of Standards for Good Practice and Outcomes in Adult Protection Work* outlines in Box 4.7 a good practice example as a training structure for staff.

**Box 4.7 Training requirements relating to vulnerable adults**

| Course | Course outline |
| --- | --- |
| **Level 1**<br>*Awareness* | Developing a shared understanding of what is abuse and what is a vulnerable adult. An understanding of the signs and symptoms of abuse. Also what to do if you witness abuse or are told about it. |
| **Level 2**<br>*The Practitioner's role* | Dealing with disclosures for those who need to complete the alert form as part of their professional role. Determining risk, vulnerability, and seriousness. Examining the implications of the three 'Cs' – capacity, consent and confidentiality. |

| Level 3 | Knowledge and skills required in planning and undertaking a protective and/or detective investigation either within a single agency or jointly with colleagues from other agencies. |
| *The Investigator's guide* | |
| | Examining elements of good practice in gathering evidence. |
| Level 4 | Developing mutual understanding of the complementary and supportive roles of the police, social services and other agencies when a potential crime has been committed. This will include an overview of the 'Achieving Best Evidence' model of interviewing. |
| *Joint working and criminal investigations* | |
| Level 5 | This course is directed at those who will be involved in the conclusive decision-making processes (such as care conferences and planning meetings) and have responsibility for these under the current policy and procedures. Evaluating the evidence and implementing protection planning. |
| *Decision making* | |
| Level 6 | Who are the stakeholders in protection planning? Providing for the post-abuse support needs of the vulnerable adult and their support networks – a strengths and needs model. Managing the impact of adult protection on the practitioners. |
| *Post-abuse* | |

*Source:* The Association of Directors of Social Services (2005: 20) *Safeguarding Adults: A National Framework of Standards for Good Practice and Outcomes in Adult Protection Work*

It is generally considered that all staff working in the NHS should have an understanding of safeguarding vulnerable adults irrespective of their individual role, be it clinical or non-clinical. This training then increases depending on whether you are expected to recognize signs of abuse, are accountable for responding, or accountable for investigating issues around safeguarding alerts.

### Child-specific training

When looking at safeguarding children and young people, we need to look at the Royal College of Paediatrics and Child Health (2010: 9) *Safeguarding Children and Young People* Intercollegiate Documents. The framework within this document describes six levels of competence (see Box 4.8) for training requirements, although it should be recognized that there will be individuals that will fall either levels above or below the recommendations; this could be because of an individual job role.

### Box 4.8 Training requirements relating to safeguarding children and young people

| Course | Target audience |
| --- | --- |
| Level 1 | Non-clinical staff working in healthcare settings |
| Level 2 | Minimum level required for clinical staff who have some degree of contact with children and young people and or parents/carers |
| Level 3 | Clinical staff working with children, young people and or their parents/carers and who could potentially contribute to assessing, planning, intervening and evaluating the needs of a child or young person and pertaining capacity where there are safeguarding/child protection concerns |
| Level 4 | Named professionals |
| Level 5 | Designated professionals |
| Level 6 | Experts |

*Source:* Royal College of Paediatrics and Child Health (2010: 9)

It is important that ODPs understand their personal responsibilities and training needs, and how this impacts on their professional accountability. ODPs should know what training is required, and should also make sure that they keep up to date with both general and departmental issues at all times.

One thing to be considered with all safeguarding initiatives is the confidentiality aspect. Patient confidentiality needs to be protected at all times, especially if told in confidence by the patient; however, we also need to think about doing the best for the patient at all times. Discussing appropriate information with a relevant manager or healthcare professional regarding the information you have received from a patient should not be thought of as a breach in confidentiality. It should be remembered that patients will feel more at ease with some individuals than with others and, as an independent registered practitioner, it is our duty to 'do no harm', whether this is this from action or omission.

**Stop and think**

Have you been in a situation where you have perceived that there has been a potential breach of patient confidentiality? How did you respond to this, and could you have done anything different?

### Learning disabilities (LD)

The ODP should also consider what impact they have on the patient experience for those individuals with an LD in the perioperative environment. The Department of Health published a Six Lives Progress Report in July 2010 that looks specifically at 'reporting on the progress made to improve care and treatment of people with learning disabilities since the publication of Six Lives'.

The Six Lives recommend that all NHS and social care organizations in England should review urgently:

- the effectiveness of the system they have in place to enable them to understand and plan to meet the full range of needs of people with learning disabilities in their areas;

and

- the capacity and capability of the service they provide and/or commission for their local populations to meet the additional and often complex needs of people with learning disabilities;

and should report according to those responsible for the governance of those organisations within 12 months of the publication of the report.

(DH, 2010: 20)

Although not an exhaustive list, some of the areas that needed to be explored include: appropriate training of staff for LD (as this is different from the vulnerable adult/child training); liaison nurse availability; and the inclusion of people with LD and their families and easy-read information.

Appropriate training should address several issues relating to LD and should include a basic understanding of LD and the differing forms this can take. Ideally, to assist with this, a member of the LD training team should have an LD of their own. The training should consider things like communication skills, the mental capacity act, consent and decision making; in addition to exploring the behavioural response to a situation, how this can be best approached and the challenges associated with it.

The role of the liaison nurse does not necessarily need to be a full-time position so would depend on the size of the individual organization. This will be someone of an appropriate grade and experience so they are able to respond appropriately to any concerns or events as and when needed. They also need to be able to communicate at Trust Board level, and then be able to feedback to all appropriate clinical and non-clinical areas.

Information should be easy to read and should not be limited to one particular area within the hospital or to a particular set of documentation. Areas for consideration are: information leaflets; are these in a format that are easy to read and in plain English, and do they need simple diagrams to support the information being discussed? Signage and whether the appropriate use of colours and images are used to distinguish different areas. The best way to make sure that these signs are appropriate for LD is to have a multidisciplinary team look at the needs of the patients and visitors. This team should include the LD liaison nurse and staff associated with the LD training team. The ideal situation would be to have a representative from the LD community to give advice on specific needs. This individual might well already be part of the LD training team.

### Stop and think

Consider whether you and your department are prepared to treat a patient with LD? If not, what can you do about it, and who would you contact to discuss any issues?

## Conclusion

This chapter has highlighted some of the aspects around patient safety in the operating theatre, why and how we should use the WHO Safe Surgery system, and how human factors can influence outcome either by individual actions, use of devices and reducing drug errors. We have also looked at why it is important to have good communication skills within the team, and why we should reduce the power gradient among members of the multidisciplinary team. We have also looked at reducing future risk by conducting an appropriate RCA as and when required. We should remember that with RCA it is not important what tool we use, but that we use it correctly. We have also highlighted training requirements around safeguarding vulnerable adults and children, and how what we do influences the care of the LD patient. We have also touched on the multi-skilled practitioner, how and why they could be used in a constantly changing NHS, but more importantly, we have discussed why this might not be best practice for all areas.

There is a real need for all aspects of human factors to be embraced within healthcare processes and education. Bromiley (2011) states that:

In the old days in Ireland if you wanted to be closer to God there were three professions: a priest, a teacher or a doctor. And the healthcare system still thinks of itself as one of those 'institutions'. It needs to shift it's thinking . . . to think like nuclear, rail, aviation or other such safety critical industries.

So, for better patient care and safer standards, the multidisciplinary team needs to embrace human factors as a way of working in professional life and make sure that it is part of the normal education process both pre- and post-registration irrespective of profession.

### Key points

- Patient safety in the operating department is a key responsibility for all members of the multidisciplinary team irrespective of job title or role.
- When completing any RCA, there should be more emphasis on completing the process correctly rather than on the complexity of the system you are using.

- All staff should be aware of appropriate policies in relation to safeguarding vulnerable adults and children.
- Staff should understand their employer's stance on LD, what provisions are in place generally, and what provisions are available within their own work area.

## References and further reading

Association of Directors of Social Services (2005) *Safeguarding Adults, A National Framework of Standards for Good Practice and Outcomes in Adult Protection Work.* London: Association of Directors of Social Services.

Aviation Knowledge (2010) *The 'Dirty Dozen' in Aviation Maintenance.* Available online at http://aviationknowledge.wikidot.com/aviation:dirty-dozen (accessed 3 February 2010).

BBC (2012) *Horizon*: Episode 10, 'Out of control', BBC2, 13 March, 2100 hours.

Bromiley, M. (2011) *Healthcare, Aviation and the Clinicians' Revolution.* Available online at http://www.health.org.uk/blog/healthcare-aviation-and-the-clinicians-revolution/ (accessed 3 February 2013).

Clinical Human Factors Group. Available online at http://www.chfg.org (accessed March 2010).

Department of Health (DH) (2010) *'Six Lives' Progress Report.* London: DH.

Department of Health (DH) (2012) *The 'Never Events' List 2012/13.* London: DH.

Federal Aviation Administration (2000) *The Human Factors Analysis and Classification System-HFACS* Available online at http://www.nifc.gov/fireinfo/fireinfo_documents/humanfactors_classanly.pdf (accessed 3 February 2013).

Flin, R., O'Conner, P. and Crichton, M. (2008) *Safety at the Sharp End.* Hampshire: Ashgate Publishing.

Lamb-Richardson, A. and Underwood, K. (2010) 'WHO, what, why and how? Safe surgery implementation', *Technic*, 1 (5): 8–9.

Medical Protection Society (2012) *Medication Errors.* Available online at http://www.medicalprotection.org/uk/booklets/common-problems-hospital/medication-errors (accessed 3 February 2013).

Risky Business (2012) *Sharing Ideas in Risk, Human Factors, Teamwork and Leadership.* Available online at http://www.risky-business.com/talk-18-story-of-bethany-bowen-2.html?channel_id=5 (accessed 3 February 2013).

Royal College of Paediatrics and Child Health (2010) *Safeguarding Children and Young People: Roles and Competencies for Health Care Staff, Intercollegiate Document.* London: Royal College of Paediatricians and Child Health.

*Safesurgery.org* (n.d.) Available online at http://www.safesurg.org (accessed 3 February 2013).

The Empowered Patient Coalition (2013) *CHFG Clinical Human Factors Group.* Available online at http://www.empoweredpatientcoalition.org/component/content/article/56-united-kingdom/228-chfg-clinical-human-factors-group (accessed 3 February 2013).

Underwood, K. (2012) 'Are you short or TALL? Reducing risk of drug errors', *Technic*, 3 (3): 6–7.

World Health Organization (WHO) (2009) *Safe Surgery Saves Lives.* Available online at www.who.int/patientsafety/safesurgery (accessed 3 March 2013).

# 5 | Psychosocial aspects of operating department practice

## *Christine Mahoney*

---

**Key topics**

- Introduction
- Why is this relevant?
- Clarification of terms
- Redefining care in health settings

- Psychosocial theories and their importance for perioperative practice
- The balance of power and control
- Psychosocial changes across the lifespan
- Stigma and the group mentality

---

## Introduction

This chapter provides an introduction to some of the theories behind people's behaviour and offers operating department practitioners (ODPs) a basis for consideration of their current practice in support and care of perioperative patients. There are a number of definitions of psychology, but it is generally considered to be a study of thought and behaviour, with the object of understanding why people behave as they do. Sociology, however, is the study of human social behaviour, focusing particularly on the organization and development of human society. Sociology looks at the ways humans interact with each other, rather than focusing specifically on the sense of self. The combination of psychology and sociology gives the phenomena of psychosocial and includes the nature of people's own behaviour, and how that behaviour may affect or be affected by interaction with others.

## Why is this relevant?

Everything that operating department practitioners (ODPs) do requires interaction with other humans, often under heightened emotional conditions and within specific time pressures. In stressful work environments it is easy to become task-oriented, which can initiate a process where patients feel (at best) *attended to* rather than *cared for*. Equally, staff-to-staff communication may become less effective under stress, and team performance will be compromised. Gaining a deeper understanding of the underpinning tenets of human behaviour will enable practitioners to appreciate what makes each person an individual, to consider current practice, and find ways to enhance interaction with all others in the theatre environment.

## Redefining care in health settings

There has been a tremendous growth in recent years of policies (both in the UK and internationally) aimed at improving 'care' of patients. These have largely emerged in response to high-profile cases reported in the media where failures in the system have led to inadequate care in various sectors of health and social care provision. At the core of every government-led inquiry into such failures is an individual human being who has suffered at the hands of those from whom they expected a satisfactory level of care, and in the process, this human being has become a statistic.

In an effort to re-establish the human context of the numerous reports, policies and protocols, it may help to reconsider what is meant by 'care' in a health setting, and in particular, in the perioperative environment.

The *Oxford Dictionary* (2010) defines care as: 'the provision of what is necessary for the health, welfare, maintenance, and protection of someone or something'. This of course could be achieved in a mechanistic, task-oriented fashion, but patients deserve more than this basic level of attention. In addition, dissatisfaction with the medical model, identified by Marks et al. (2005), supports the argument for a more holistic, person-centred attitude to care in health. A level of care that involves supporting someone through their own understanding of their diagnosis and treatment requires acknowledgement of the patient as an individual, with complex behavioural attributes based on previous experience and upbringing. The psychosocial approach recognizes the ways that human experience, culture and society influence our attitudes to health. The World Health Organization (WHO, 1946) defined health as 'a state of complete physical, mental and social well-being and not merely the absence of disease', and although this view of health has been challenged with a change in the pattern of disease during the interim half century, mental and social wellbeing must still form a central ideal in healthcare. People experience the National Health Service (NHS) at times of basic human need, when care and compassion are what matter most (Department of Health (DH), 2012). Patients feel that shortfalls in care, impersonal treatment and lack of compassion reveal a lack of respect on the part of the practitioner.

In a busy operating theatre department, care of the patient has as many components that will be delivered by a number of multidisciplinary staff. The ODP must ensure safe positioning, checking equipment, maintaining infection control, acting as a patient advocate and ensuring accurate recording of events that all contribute to the care of a surgical patient. However, if the individual receiving such care does not feel the ODP is compassionate, an opportunity to improve the patient experience has been lost.

### Stop and think

Consider the department you work in. Have you ever observed where the individual has received impersonal or offhand treatment? Might this have happened when a patient is behaving 'differently' or is 'not communicating'?

## Psychological theories and their importance for perioperative practice

Psychology, broadly speaking, is an attempt to explain why people behave as they do. Why does behaviour vary significantly between individuals faced with the same situation or, for that matter, why might a person behave differently in different circumstances?

### What is a 'psychological theory'?

Psychologists have, over many years, developed a number of 'approaches' to the subject, and within each of these approaches (or perspectives) there are equally as many individual theories. In each case the theorist presents an argument as to why a person may exhibit particular behaviour. Some theories are widely accepted, others hotly contested, and there is no conclusive evidence for any one of the specific approaches. Indeed, trying to analyse an individual's behaviour from only one psychological perspective would be impossible – humans are far too complex for that.

This broad range of explanations may lead the reader to deduce that none of the theories are accurate since they cannot be proved or disproved. From a purely scientific perspective, nothing is ever proved, and all findings remain theories until such times as further evidence can challenge their accuracy. Taking the psychologist's viewpoint, the theories give a position from which to debate and discuss observable human phenomena.

It is difficult to imagine now that there was a time when these subjects were not the topic of debate – when no one considered it necessary to analyse behaviour or offer explanations for it. The various studies of the mind, and subsequent development of theories, have given people the vocabulary and the framework to talk about and understand human behaviour in a way that is now taken for granted. Thoughts or feelings may be described as 'subconscious' or 'unconscious', with a sound expectation that others will know what this means. A person may be described as having a 'complex', and people will understand how that affects behaviour, yet these words were unheard of in this context until the latter part of the nineteenth century.

The following psychological approaches will be considered against observable behaviour in the operating department and is intended only to encourage the reader to broaden their understanding of basic psychological processes as may be apparent in the perioperative environment.

## The psychodynamic approach to psychology and the Freudian perspective

The psychodynamic approach relates to a number of theories that consider what drives or motivates humans in their behaviour, and in particular the effects initiated by the unconscious mind. Sigmund Freud (1856–1939) remains the most influential psychodynamic theorist. Freud's psychoanalytic theory relies on the observation that human behaviour has its roots in early childhood experiences – often experiences that we are unable to consciously remember. Perhaps most famously Freud postulated that the unconscious mind may be divided into three basic areas – the *id*, the *ego* and the *superego*. Tensions between these three factions can cause anxiety, and people therefore develop coping or defence mechanisms that can be observed.

The 'id' is associated with basic, primal, innate instincts, associated principally with survival. According to Bruce and Borg (2002) Freud coined the term lib-id-o meaning 'vital energy', although it has since come to be associated solely with sexual instincts. Freud's explanation of the id includes sexual instincts, but also covers aggression associated with self-protection, and he proposed the id was incapable of logical thought.

The 'superego' responds to the morals and rules of society – what some people refer to as the mind's conscience. This area is thought to develop around the ages of three to six years, and is what governs the ways we 'ought' to behave in society. The superego's role is to contain the desires of the id by observing the rules of society, and this can create tensions.

If the ODP was to consider these in respect to a surgical patient, the self-preserving id will want to run away from this terrifying experience of allowing strangers to undertake procedures from which the body may not recover. The superego will be forcing the individual to 'behave nicely' in this situation because the staff are there to help, and it is not acceptable to make a fuss. These competing reactions can start a cycle of mutually reinforcing events of aggressive self-protection and embarrassment at inappropriate behaviour. This increases anxiety within a patient who will already be feeling self-conscious due to a number of other factors including nudity, fear of the unknown and possibly needle or other phobias.

The third of Freud's proposed sections of the mind is the 'ego' that attempts to mediate between the id and the superego to find a balance. It does this by storing up previously experienced responses to specific stimuli, and producing an appropriate response to deal with a specific tension. The ego recognizes the tensions between innate, self-preservation instincts and the need to conform to society's rules, and employs a number of defence or coping mechanisms in its role as mediator. Examples of these coping strategies are clearly observable in perioperative patients, therefore the ODP needs to identify and respond to these:

- Denial – the patient may be unable to engage in discussion about the procedure or associated interventions. Therefore, the ODP needs to be aware of the signs for example the inability to maintain eye contact or focusing on repetitive actions (e.g. folding and unfolding a tissue or plucking at the sheet).
- Displacement – becoming angry with others not necessarily involved in the immediate process. For example, blaming the ward staff for not explaining things properly, or declaiming the actions of whoever the patient may see as responsible for their being in hospital (the government, the nuclear industry, the cat that they fell over, etc.).
- Regression – retreating to childhood behaviours that are seen as comforting; for example, thumb-sucking, or rocking back and forth with their arms wrapped around them.
- Reaction formation – behaviours that would normally be considered a sign of weakness or inappropriate; for example, crying, are substituted by the opposite behaviour such as overconfidence or exceptionally chatty.

### Stop and think

Freud's theories can equally be applied to staff as well as patients. Can you think of examples where a colleague's behaviour may be explained according to the psychoanalytic approach? What might be provoking the id, and what might the ego be initiating to mediate the behaviour?

Freud's theories have been challenged by many as being too reductionist, trying to predict behaviour of a whole species based on close examination of a few individuals. The abstract nature of his concept of self has also been questioned, but since the behaviours he described are evidently portrayed in people under stress, the approach may be seen as relevant and believable to those involved in healthcare.

### The behaviourist approach – reinforcement and conditioning

Another psychological approach is behaviourism, founded by John Watson in 1913 (and later expanded by B.F. Skinner) with its roots in Pavlovian response theory. In direct contrast to Freud's introspective approach (looking at internal, abstract phenomena) the behaviourist approach is concerned with observable reactions to specific external stimuli, and this approach dominated psychology for the first half of the twentieth century. Watson believed that personality develops as a result of learned behaviours, which are mostly influenced by others and the environment. As such, he suggested that objective scientific studies on stimulus and response could be undertaken, which would allow predictions to be made about behaviour in defined circumstances.

The behaviourist approach discounts internal personal motivation, and focuses instead on stimulus–response interactions that have come to be known as 'conditioning'. Pavlov's famous experiment that demonstrated dogs salivating whenever the idea of food was presented to them – not just once they actually saw the food – led to further studies on conditioned responses.

Conditioning happens because specific responses are repeatedly experienced in association with the same stimuli, and can be positive or negative in association. In positive terms, a person may be more inclined to undertake a particular process because previous experience suggests a pleasurable outcome. Perhaps due to scepticism, positive conditioning tends to be less evident than negative conditioning, where scenarios may be avoided because in the past they have caused pain or stress.

Upton (2012) describes a phenomenon known as anticipatory nausea and vomiting (ANV) where patients undergoing chemotherapy for cancer would report nausea and/or vomiting prior to the chemotherapy drugs being administered. Such is the power of classical conditioning; patients would begin to feel nauseous on entering the ward, or even when they attend the same hospital for another matter.

Negative reinforcement seems to be harder to challenge than positive reinforcement, and even if the stimulus does not produce the expected response, it takes a long while for the learned behaviour to subside. For example, a person may develop a needle phobia because of only one unpleasant experience. Any subsequent painless injections or cannulations would be viewed as exceptions or 'flukes', and would not change the anticipatory behaviour of fear and withdrawal. Of course, fear initiates the stress response and actually contributes to a negative experience, so a negative association cycle is particularly difficult to break.

### Stop and think

How might hospital induced anxiety be explained according to conditioning theory? Is there anything you could do as an ODP to alleviate the stress associated with the experience in the perioperative environment?

Associated with the conditioning described above is the related concept of operant conditioning, whereby the individual has a role to play in influencing the outcome. That is to say, by exhibiting particular behaviours, a positive response (or reward) may be elicited.

Clearly, a real change in behaviour requires repeated exposure to the stimulus–reward concept. This may not be practicable within theatres due to the infrequent nature of the patient interactions, but an understanding of this process may enable the ODP to appreciate how their own behaviour may influence future patient experiences. If, due to staff shortages or the pressure of a busy list, a practitioner fails to take time to give a patient their undivided attention, the patient's sense of being a nuisance or a bother will be reinforced. This might mean that in future a patient fails to divulge something of importance when questioned. Conversely, putting the patient at the centre of the therapeutic relationship will enhance feelings of trust and importance, which could make future experiences less upsetting.

Expectancy that a particular behaviour may elicit the same response in the future, based on past experience, is a learning theory proposed by Albert Bandura (1977), which is based on the behaviourist approach. Bandura indicated that people with a low expectancy (of reward) will put little effort into changing their behaviour. This low expectancy is often influenced by the subjective observation of behaviour in others, as well as past experience of one's own perceived ability to change (e.g. 'I can't lose weight no matter how I try – my mother was just the same.').

This can be seen in what we call 'vicariously learned' attitudes; for example, children learn by observation of their parents'/carers' behaviour. If a child sees that their mother or father is anxious about a visit to hospital, and that such a visit results in pain to the parent, then the child will be anxious that the same response will result for them. This phenomenon is not unique to children, the response may become further reinforced throughout the lifespan, resulting in adults who are still anxious or fearful based on the behaviour of their parents some 30 years before.

**Stop and think**

How much of your professional behaviour is influenced by 'vicariously' learned attitudes from your peers? Do you find yourself changing your behaviour depending on who you are working with? Do you ever find yourself using this as an excuse for your own behaviour?

Cognitive psychology evolved from the behaviourist approach, and focused on the mechanistic processing of thought, based on the impersonal logic-based flow diagrams now familiar with computer programmers. Much of the research into cognitive psychology relies on scientific, laboratory-based experiments, and as such attracts criticism as real life is not like a laboratory. The lack of the personal, emotional element in the various theories within behaviourism encouraged a break away from this perspective to an approach that puts the human condition at the centre of the studies.

### The humanist approach, and the influence of identity

The humanist or person-centred approach was developed as a reaction to the previous dominant themes in psychology. Based on the work of Abraham Maslow (1970) and Carl Rogers (1951), these theories focus on the emotional and physical needs of the human condition, and the concept of 'self'. In humanist terms, the personal nature of human experience including love, creativity, hope, health, individuality and value are all components that add to the complexity of human behaviour. Both Maslow and Rogers firmly believed that people have a natural tendency to move towards health, growth and positive self-concept, assuming the right conditions are present.

Maslow developed a model demonstrating how people will naturally move towards emotional and cognitive fulfilment, providing their basic 'life needs' are met. In simple terms, deficiency in any of the basic elements of human need (food, shelter, safety, love, respect) will prevent a person from achieving their full potential, or 'self-actualization'. The human psyche, one might say, is concerned with self-preservation and recognition of its own value, above any other less vital concerns such as intelligence or beauty. When the whole human condition is under threat, for example, during illness, then often the lower-level needs to take complete precedence (food, sleep and attention) and higher concerns such as personal attractiveness are ignored.

Rogers agreed with Maslow, but concluded that a person could not achieve this personal growth alone as they needed positive reinforcement from those around them in the form of genuineness, acceptance and empathy. He also made it clear that each person is unique – that they each have their own 'pinnacle' of achievement, which will not be the same as anyone else, even someone who had encountered exactly the same environmental and emotional conditions. The sense of 'self' or identity – what makes each of us exactly what we are – is central to Rogers' theory of person-centred psychology.

In healthcare terms, this means in order to care effectively for an individual, the ODP needs to take some time to determine what it is that a person needs, not to make assumptions based on what would make the practitioner feel better in the same situation. How often has the phrase 'treat patients as you would wish to be treated' been passed on from practitioner to learner? In Rogers' terms this should be rephrased – treat the patient as *they* would wish to be treated.

Rogers' concept of self includes two separate identities – actual self (the person as they really are) and ideal self (the person they would like to be). If these two entities are vastly different, the person would feel uncomfortable experiencing low self-esteem and lacking in confidence. In order to balance the two entities a person requires permission (or positive regard) from those around them, even if they behave in a 'less than ideal' fashion.

If the ODP was to apply this to the perioperative patient, the perception of actual self (anxious, helpless, a nuisance, unable to deal with the situation) will likely be far removed from their ideal self (confident, grown up, in control), and this will manifest itself in what might be termed 'disordered' behaviour. This could result in anxiety certainly or possibly aggression, rudeness or even withdrawal. For the ODP to be able to support patients in this position, the patient must perceive a genuine interest in their welfare rather than an 'adopted' professional attitude, and the ODP needs to develop these skills. The patient will need acceptance, empathy and above all 'congruent' or genuine communication. This means that words are not enough, the practitioner's body language and personal attention need to reinforce the therapeutic nature of the communication.

**Stop and think**

Think about a situation you have encountered in the perioperative environment recently where someone's behaviour appeared bizarre or 'unacceptable'. In the light of your understanding of psychological approaches, can you now offer explanations for why they behaved this way, and how the situation might have been handled better?

## Psychosocial theories and their importance for perioperative practice

Psychological theories can help explain the behaviour of an individual, but it is recognized that social factors such as the environment, culture and peer pressure can also impact on behaviour. People do not live or behave in isolation, and the context of the social setting within which people function has an effect on behaviour. The term 'psychosocial' has evolved, which seeks to explore and explain the influence of these external factors. Psychosocial theories focus on the premise that the human character is fundamentally social in nature, and how an individual relates to others shapes their personality. Many theories (Heinz Kohut, Karen Horney) focus on early social interactions with parents and carers, which are thought to give a grounding to a wider social application in later life.

However, Erik Erikson (1902–1994) considered that personality development continued throughout life into adulthood, and utilized a 'staged' model of development, with each stage representing a crisis that had to be resolved before the individual could move on to the next stage. Largely speaking, Erikson's theory focuses on the individual finding the solutions to these crises by interacting with others, rather than being the passive recipient of attention.

As it is widely accepted that behaviour is intrinsically linked with surroundings and social circle, it is self-evident that changing the social structure of the environment will affect behaviour in some way. When considering the behaviour of patients, not only must one make allowance about what might be considered 'normal' for them in their own socio-cultural setting, one must also recognize that for the duration of the therapeutic relationship, the society in which they find themselves (the hospital) is alien and therefore outside the normative rules that they find comfortable.

**Stop and think**

What aspects of societal behaviour are considered normal in a hospital setting that would not be acceptable in other areas of life? (If you are finding this difficult, think perhaps about the routine questions we ask patients – 'Do you have any false teeth?' or 'When did you last have a bowel movement?')

### How does environment impact on the patient's ability to cope?

Erving Goffman (1968) did a considerable amount of work on the effect institutions had on personality (or 'the self' as he described it). His work identified similarities between the populations of prisons and mental hospitals, and he suggested that the culture of institutions had a specific effect on the people who lived within them. His view was that institutions change people, and he also warned that the conditions that make prisons 'prisonlike' can be found in many other institutions where the residents have broken no laws.

The impact of rituals and hierarchical management structures on individual behaviour can, to a greater or lesser extent, be applied to patients undergoing hospital treatment, and specifically to most theatre patients. In Goffman's terms, the features of an institution include: the processing or treatment of individuals; a clear distinction between inmates (patients) and staff; and the segregation of those under the care of the institution from wider society. All of these criteria are applicable to the perioperative environment at some level, and therefore the dehumanizing or depersonalization of those subjected to this false society is not difficult to identify.

The effect that Goffman proposes is discussed extensively by Lee and Newby (1983) who describe the term *disculturation* as a progressive process by which the minutiae of the person's pre-admission self are gradually eroded, in order to leave a personality that will be submissive to the requirements of the institution.

It may not be comfortable to view the standard preoperative processes in this way – the processes are, after all, there for a reason (e.g. removing outdoor clothes, wearing a standard issue hospital gown, being shaved, removing dentures, glasses or hearing aid) but the effect on the self will be the same, whatever the reason for implementing the process. Add to this the violation of personal space – by medical examination, or even just by the application of ECG electrodes or a blood pressure cuff – and assigning patients a number, which is checked against a list, over and over again, it soon becomes evident how effectively routine behaviour can reduce even the most well-balanced personality to a non-person.

The ODP can unwittingly reinforce the norms of institutionalized behaviour when confronted with a busy list and the demands of a pressured theatre team. Unless the staff are vigilant, the relentless conveyor-belt nature of some theatre lists can surreptitiously influence the nature of patient communication to the point of mechanized responses. Sarafino (2008) describes this as a phenomenon whereby staff act as if the person had dropped their body off at the repair shop and would return for it later – a phenomenon in which some patients may appear complicit by the nature of their withdrawal from the reality of the situation.

## The balance of power and control

The changes in accepted societal behaviour in a hospital setting mean healthcare practitioners have an implicit power over the people in their care, which should not be underestimated. Blaber (2012) counsels that practitioners must be mindful of the potential to abuse this power. Society is based on unwritten rules of behaviour requiring congruence of roles and responsibilities. Goffman (1990) addressed this concept of society using the analogy of a performance, with the cast taking on specific roles and co-operating together in a performance team.

### How do professional roles 'play out' in the operating department?

Goffman suggests that a profession's public image may depend on props or costumes, which mark them out as having particular roles – consider how theatre blues, masks, stethoscopes, and so on identify a member of the theatre team. At the same time, specific behaviour is expected of people who are wearing the costumes and using the props. The way in which a theatre team behaves when setting up for a morning list, with light-hearted banter and conversation, undergoes a seamless transition into professional mode when the patient enters. From this point the anaesthetist becomes 'Dr Jones' (when normally everyone would call him Dave), and this expresses to the patient that there is professional respect within the team. As Goffman would assert; 'Backstage familiarity is suppressed' (Goffman, 1990: 166).

This effectively places the patient in the position of the audience to this team performance. However, other sources describe the ease with which patients fall into the role expected of them in a hospital setting. Sarafino (2008) suggests that the environment encourages patients to believe their involvement in their care is irrelevant – that people *learn* to be helpless in hospital. He discusses the concept whereby staff view compliant or passive patients as 'good', while unco-operative or challenging patients are regarded as a problem. A patient who is severely ill may be forgiven for being difficult, but patients who complain despite not necessarily suffering significantly may be regarded as troublemakers. Patients who are labelled as difficult may then perceive they get treated with less compassion than they deserve. Whether this actually happens does not necessarily change the perception (see *conditioning* on pp. 70–72). Patients do not want to antagonize busy staff, or be thought of as a nuisance, and therefore accept a submissive role in co-operation with the staff.

Inadvertently, the performance of the professional team underpins the hierarchical difference between the (important) staff and the (lowly) patient (from the patient's perspective), especially if what follows reinforces the imbalance of power in the relationship. By necessity, the patient will be the passive recipient of actions by the staff; that is, he will require having procedures 'done to him'. This is counter-intuitive to the basic human preservation instinct and needs to be handled sensitively.

Patients have expectations about how staff will behave in a therapeutic encounter. Staff need to comply with the positive aspects of those expectations (professional, compassionate, knowledgeable) without reinforcing the behaviours that carry a negative connotation (overbearing, patronizing, overfamiliar, inappropriately jovial), in order to make the patient feel as comfortable as possible. Learners in the perioperative environment need to identify which members of the team demonstrate these attributes most effectively, and work towards emulating effective patient communication. Defining such behaviour, or explaining why one member of staff can apparently say and do exactly the same as another with very different results, requires understanding of the complex nature of human interaction. Extending Goffman's theatrical analogy, having the right cast and the right script *may* result in a believable performance, or may equally result in a catastrophic medley of unconvincing characters and bad acting. In order to produce a believable performance the cast members need to *inhabit* the characters completely, to *be* the professional, not to *act* the professional. This will then enhance the congruence of genuine communication, discussed earlier (see *humanist* approach on p. 72).

The way in which an ODP performs their professional role will change within given parameters, depending on the interaction they experience with the individual patient. Of course, there has to be a baseline of accepted professional behaviour, but the circumstances of the relationship and the needs of the individual cannot help but affect the outcome of the performance. Flexibility is the key here, and learning to interpret the nuances of the patient's communication is paramount. The aim of any interaction with a patient must surely be to achieve a given purpose for the patient, not to generate a feeling of satisfaction or self-importance in the practitioner.

**Stop and think**

Can you identify instances where you or a colleague may have behaved in a particular way to impress a senior member of staff, without necessarily considering how that behaviour may have looked to the patient?

Despite advances in patients' rights, there is still an accepted belief among patients that they need to co-operate with the professionals who are looking after them. Implicitly, this allows the practitioner to exercise power over the patient, because the patient is aware of the need to comply with requests made in what they believe will be their best interests.

### The nature of power in the therapeutic relationship

Power, in and of itself, is a complex entity to comprehend, leading to a general acceptance of it being dependent on principles of domination and exploitation. Traditionally, power is presented as an object that can be held – or lost. However, the philosopher Michel Foucault (1926–1984) presented a counter-argument about how power works, which suggests that it is relative rather than concrete, that it is not a structure, but a strategy, and that it cannot be held, it can only be exercised. Foucault's suggestion (Gauntlett, 2008) is that power requires context, and a person who is able to exercise power (not *hold* power) in one setting; for example, the chief executive officer (CEO) of a successful company is not necessarily perceived as powerful in another setting. Foucault asserts that power does not exist outside social relationships, but within relationships it is evident at every level.

Upton (2012) discusses power in the framework of relationships, suggesting it is the extent to which an individual can persuade another person to act in a certain way. Upton explains that there are various types of persuasive technique that individuals may exploit to influence another's behaviour, and of these, *expert power*, where one party has greater knowledge than the other, is evidently applicable to the practitioner–patient relationship. If Foucault's model of power relies on reciprocal tacit agreement between the two parties, then the balance of power can be altered, by changing the level of control held by each. It is unlikely that a patient will actively try to take control, due to the multifaceted psychological and psychosocial principles outlined above, which lead him to accept the need for compliance and co-operation. In an operating theatre setting, the *powerful experts* are able to exert total control over the patient's existence in the immediate future, and that is accepted. However, the ODP has the capacity to restore the balance by releasing control and gifting the power back to the patient. This is a challenging concept; practitioners are not intentionally wielding power over another, weaker, individual, but simply by performing their role they may be creating tensions within patients who experience the very real powerlessness of surrendering to the actions of the healthcare practitioners.

Foucault suggests that where power exists, resistance is inevitable, and such resistance may be evident as 'quiet tensions and suppressed concern, or spontaneous anger' (Gauntlett, 2008: 131). These manifestations mirror the coping strategies of denial and displacement identified by Freud when the id and the superego are in opposition.

The practitioner needs to consider whether their communication style is profession-centred or person-centred, and where this places the power in the relationship. For example:

'Hello, My name is Jim and I shall be looking after you today. I just need to check your name band, [picks up arm, reads . . .], 5734628, thank you. Now, I have to attach these various machines to you, so that we can keep an eye on all your vital signs while we've got you here today . . .'

Most practitioners can identify with these words. On the face of it, the words are friendly, and meet the requirement of keeping the patient informed of what is going on. On closer examination, however, the power is all focused on the professional 'I' am going to do all these things to 'you' and 'you' just have to put up with it.

By reframing the conversation to put the patient at the centre, the power can be handed back to the patient:

'Hello Mrs Jones, you are our first patient today. I'm Jim, and my job is to make sure you are comfortable and cared for while you are with us. Although we need to check a few details with you, I want you to know you can ask us about anything that you are unsure of, and if you feel uncomfortable about anything you just have to say and we'll do all we can to make things feel better. Do you mind if I attach these ECG electrodes and blood pressure cuff? Which arm is more comfortable for you?'

Of course, the material outcome is the same; the patient gets checked in, necessary procedures are carried out, requirements are met, and in effect the patient is still at the mercy of the practitioner and the procedure. However the psychological impact on the patient in the second example is far lower than the first. Restoring the power, even notionally, to the patient and thereby reducing resistance (consciously or unconsciously) should have a positive effect both on the current procedure, and any future encounters with the perioperative team.

### Stop and think

Rehearse one of your recent patient conversations, and consider how the power balance was being influenced by your actions. Could you change the way you approach these conversations to empower patients more effectively?

## Psychosocial changes across the lifespan

Much of what has been written so far in this chapter has related to the care of 'a patient', and can, at first principles, be applied to the care of patients across the lifespan. Generally, when considering patient care in theatres, the patient is taken to be an adult, although because that could cover any person over the age of 18, there is going to be a considerable difference in cognitive, experiential and intellectual ability across patients even in this category. At the same time, placing patients in an unfamiliar environment, under stressful and emotional conditions is very likely to result in behaviour that may not be considered 'age appropriate'. For this reason it is not helpful to categorize patients as possessing specific psychosocial attributes at the various stages of their lifespan, this leads to group definitions that are both unhelpful and (at their core) discriminatory (see *Stigma and the group mentality* on p. 79).

Both cognitive and psychosocial development is a continuous process across the lifespan, and human responses will depend on the internal experiential resources available to the patient at the time of their surgery. Of course, there are developmental differences across the stages of the lifespan, perhaps most famously described by Erik Erikson, but it must be accepted that the boundaries between these stages are not distinct, and that not every patient will exhibit these behaviours at any particular stage of their life.

Erikson's theory is based on Freud's psychoanalytical approach, although he does not completely agree with Freud's model. In Erikson's opinion, individual and societal development is a cyclical process, continually affecting and being affected one by the other. Every personal and social 'crisis' gives an individual experience, which will contribute to that individual's emotional or psychological growth. The crises that Erikson describes relate to polar-opposite forces that simultaneously challenge humans: on the one hand to strive, grow, reach out for new experiences; on the other hand to retreat to a place of lesser complexity and, by definition, greater comfort (Maier, 1978). In Erikson's view, these crises require resolving in order for a human being to achieve fulfilment, and broadly speaking behaviour at different points of the lifespan is associated with different conflicts.

Erikson considers that a person is not a static product of their upbringing, that they are constantly people 'under construction', capable of constantly developing and redeveloping, and he describes eight stages of personality development. For example, the earliest conflict is trust versus mistrust, which relates to babies in their first year. For the newborn, a sense of trust requires a feeling of physical comfort, with a minimum amount of uncertainty. Mistrust will arise from unsatisfactory physical experiences (hunger, abandonment, etc.) and frustration that may lead in later years to apprehension. The next stage, between one and three years of age is concerned with developing autonomy versus doubt and shame. Children of this age start to want to make their own decisions and take control of their life and struggle with the need to develop autonomy, but recognize this behaviour may alienate them from their carers and ultimately leave them defenceless.

### General principles for dealing with young people

Caring for paediatric patients in the perioperative environment requires the ODP to have the fundamental understanding that children are not just small adults. Children do not process information logically or rationally in the same way that adults can, even in familiar and relaxed environments. Hospitalization, and the journey to theatres, presents children with situations that in their home life would be seen as dangerous, frightening and disruptive. They are expected to talk to strangers, to agree to situations that appear uncomfortable and out of their control. Even though most paediatric patients are accompanied to theatres by their parents or primary carer, the emotional toll on those adults creates tensions that the children further fail to understand. Why is mummy crying? Why is daddy scared?

The key to caring for paediatric patients is the co-operation of the whole perioperative team, and recognition that operating theatre lists may not be completed on time. This is because the approach required to receive, check in and anaesthetize children for surgery successively depends on proceeding at a pace that *the child* finds comfortable. Forcing a child to undergo clinical interventions such as cannulation or gaseous induction because the needs of the list are pressing is unacceptable in the same way, and for the same reasons, that using physical chastisement as a punishment is unacceptable in today's society (Martin, 2010).

From a power perspective, allowing children the opportunity to make their own choices (within carefully thought out parameters) allows the acknowledgement of autonomy. Providing the parameters are suitably identified in advance; it makes little difference to the perioperative team whether the child chooses option A or option B, but the psychological advantage of giving control of the situation to the patient will pay dividends. Once the child has invested in the situation by contributing to the decision making, they will then be more likely to want active involvement in the process.

Gaining a child's trust is paramount, and this requires careful handling of the interaction between clinical staff, the primary carer and the patient. Different approaches are required, which ostensibly have nothing whatsoever to do with the task in hand. Being able to discuss the relative merits of children's television programmes, or identify characters in the toys that may be accompanying the child to theatres is a good tactic, but only if it is tackled with sincerity. One thing children are adept at is identifying subterfuge and distraction techniques – they have had plenty of experience of being manipulated by parents keen to encourage specific behaviours by bribery or clever questioning!

### Things to consider for older adults

At the other end of the lifespan, elderly patients often suffer the indignity of being treated like children, no matter what level of respect they may have commanded throughout their adult life. Age is often described as being nothing more than a state of mind; however, Kastenbaum (1979) distinguishes between chronological age, biological age, subjective and functional age, which account for the differences in psychological outlook associated with increasing years. As a person ages, their health requirements (biological age) may dictate an increasing dependence on others to care for their physical needs. The loss of independence – or in psychological terms the loss of 'self' – can impact upon the person in a number of ways, including loss of identity and decreasing self-worth.

Patients who can recognize their increasing reliance on others fear becoming a nuisance or a burden, which effectively compounds their loss of engagement with, and usefulness to, society. This may result in a gradual removal of the person from societal and emotional fulfilment. The fact that this time of life often coincides with the person's increasing need for hospital treatment can exacerbate the psychological difficulties that they are experiencing.

Caring for elderly patients, especially in the perioperative environment, may require strategies to deal with deteriorating physical faculties. Poor vision, poor hearing and lack of mobility will be evident in many patients. Reduced cognitive abilities may be present, and the incidence of dementia (which is associated with, but not restricted to, patients who fall into the older-adult age bracket) is growing across the world. Often patients suffering with dementia become angry and frustrated at their inability to make sense of everyday situations, and therefore stressful encounters with healthcare practitioners are likely to produce extreme behaviour. While compassion, patience and positive regard may be considered important for all patients, these attributes are paramount when dealing with patients who have lost their in-built psychosocial compass due to the dehumanizing effects of dementia.

## Stigma and the group mentality

Earlier in the chapter, Goffman's theories about team performance provided an analogy that helped to explain patient and staff roles. Goffman (1990) also indicated that backstage the performers (i.e. the theatre staff) often refer to members of the audience using terms that would not be used in face-to-face communication. He suggests a code title may be used that categorizes the audience member (patient) in some way. It is not unusual to hear a patient being descried as 'the hernia', 'the emergency' or 'the drug user', without this necessarily representing a lack of respect for the individual per se. It is a practice that arises out of custom or habit, rather than intended malice, but does not take account of what makes each of the patients labelled in this way different from each other.

Marks et al. (2005) suggest that when people are perceived to possess attributes that lead to them being treated differently they are said to be stigmatized. The stigma could be a deformity, a disease, an undesirable social history, or because of class, nationality or creed. The word stigma comes from the ancient Greek and means a mark or brand on the skin – literally, people who are 'marked out' as different.

Despite advances in legislation preventing discrimination based on a person's background or lifestyle choices, and the implementation of professional ethics that stipulate the need to treat everyone with equal respect, it is still evident that some practitioners consider care requirements in group categories. The habitual labelling of patients with coded titles described above may lead to a more widespread 'group mentality' where the practitioner anticipates patients' care needs according to some aspect of their persona that marks them apart from the norm. For example, the stigma of 'special needs', 'high risk' or 'elderly' is inappropriate, and demonstrates an inability to recognize the differences that make each person unique.

### Stop and think

What assumptions do you make about patients when setting up for a theatre list? Do you try to avoid certain theatre sessions that you perceive will present particularly difficult patients? Do you see this as discrimination?

## Conclusion

The focus on the psychological and psychosocial theories should help to explain the complexities of human behaviour, in general terms and with specific reference to perioperative care. It should provide ODPs with a foundation for appreciating the breadth of experiences that individual patients bring to the perioperative environment. This chapter has discussed the common behaviours that may be exhibited by people coming to theatres, and highlighted similarities in human experience under specific circumstances. An understanding of these similarities requires a simultaneous acknowledgement of difference. Individuals all bring their own specific baggage to any situation, which may be similar to others in the same context, but this must not be assumed. Clearly, it is not possible to know everything about a patient prior to their hospital visit, and common procedures will follow prescribed patterns for all patients. A skilful ODP will be able to adapt, through effective communication skills and recognition of the conflicts facing the patient, in order to deliver effective, compassionate care that meets the needs of the individual.

**Key points**

- Patients will be affected by their psychological drivers.
- The application of key psychosocial theories to the perioperative environment.
- How hospital can change the way people behave, resulting in psychological conflict.
- ODPs should be aware of the power balance and understand why this should be handed back to the patient whenever possible.
- Patients should be treated as individuals.

**References and further reading**

Bandura, A. (1977) *Social Learning Theory*. Upper Saddle River, NJ: Prentice Hall.

Blader, A. (2012) 'Psychosocial aspects of health and illness an introduction', in Blader, A. (ed.) *Foundations for Paramedic Practice: A Theoretical Perspective*. Maidenhead: Open University Press.

Bruce, M. and Borg, B. (2002) *Psychosocial Frames of Reference: Core for Occupation Based Practice* (3rd edn). Thorofare, NJ: Slack Publications.

Department of Health (DH) (2012) *The NHS Constitution for England*. London: DH. Available online at www.dh.gov.uk/en/Publicationsandstatistics/Publications/PublicationsPolicyAndGuidance/DH_132961

Gauntlett, D. (2008) *Media, Gender and Identity: An Introduction* (2nd edn). London: Routledge.

Goffman, E. (1990) *The Presentation of Self in Everyday Life*. Harmondsworth: Penguin.

Goffman, E. (1968) *Asylums: Essays on the Social Situations of Mental Patients and Other Inmates*. Harmondsworth: Penguin.

Kastenbaum, R. (1979) *Growing Old: Years of Fulfillment*. London: Harper & Row.

Kohut, H. (2009) *The Restoration of the Self*. London: University of Chicago Press.

Lee, D. and Newby, H. (1983) *The Problem with Sociology*. London: Hutchinson.

Maier, H. (1978) *Three Theories of Child Development*. New York: Harper & Row.

Marks, D.F., Murray, M., Evans, B., Willig, C., Sykes, C. and Woodall, C. (2005) *Health Psychology, Theory, Research and Practice* (2nd edn). London: Sage Publications.

Martin, R. (2010) *POEMS Course Online Forum*. Available online at http://www.poemsforchildren.us/forum/index.php

Maslow, A. (1970) *Motivation and Personality* (2nd edn). New York: Harper & Row.

*Oxford Dictionary* (2010) Available online at http://oxforddictionaries.com/definition/english/care

Rogers, C. (1951) *Client-centered Therapy: Its Current Practice, Implications and Theory*. London: Constable.

Sarafino, E. (2008) *Health Psychology: Biopsychosocial Interractions* (6th edn). Hoboken, NJ: John Wiley & Sons, Inc.

Upton, D. (2012) *Introducing Psychology for Nurses and Healthcare Professionals* (2nd edn). Harlow: Pearson.

World Health Organization (WHO) (1946) *Preamble to the Constitution of the World Health Organization as Adopted by the International Health Conference*. New York: WHO.

# 6 | Legal frameworks for Operating Department Practitioners

## Helen Booth

---

**Key topics**

- Introduction
- Why this is relevant
- Understanding of civil and criminal law
- Legal statutes in relation to professional practice

- Consent
- Confidentiality
- Whistle blowing
- Conscientious objection in participation of treatment

---

## Introduction to the law

The aim of this chapter is to give the Operating Department Practitioner (ODP) a broad understanding of the legal issues that affect their practice. It is not exhaustive and, due to the complexities of many of the relevant pieces of law, it is recommended that the ODP should access the references given to gain a more in-depth understanding.

The law applies to all individuals, though professionals are named where there are specific requirements for them. One good example of this is the Misuse of Drugs and Misuse of Drugs (Safe Custody) regulations amendment 2007 where ODPs are specifically mentioned to give clarity to the safe handling of controlled drugs.

This chapter explores pertinent legislation relevant to ODPs, and discuss the impact that it has specifically for the ODP. It will also use, as appropriate, examples and discussion points but these are not exhaustive and you should relate the content to your own experiences wherever possible.

English law is concerned with two distinctive systems – civil and criminal law. The law derives from the judgments of the courts (common law) or from the legislative work of Parliament. Legislation can vary in the UK but generally these are defined into England and Wales, Northern Ireland and Scotland. Therefore, the ODP needs to be aware of any variation in the legal systems for each respective country where they are working.

## Why this is relevant

ODPs work in a high-risk area where patients are at their most vulnerable. A sound understanding of responsibility, accountability and the legal parameters of their role is therefore essential. The law described in this chapter varies in terms of how it impacts on the individual practitioner. More advanced roles bring a greater degree of depth and scope of understanding in relation to specific legislation and again the practitioner needs to be aware of this. It is paramount that the ODP accesses current legislation through government websites. ODPs should, as part of their continual development, access these websites to update themselves and to reflect how these may impact on their practice. There is no excuse for ignorance with regard to adhering to legal requirements related to the ODP role.

## Understanding the differences of civil and criminal law

*Civil law* governs the relationship between the individual and state organizations and covers a vast array of areas. In the context of health, the focus will be on the civil law of tort. Tort is the area of law concerned with 'remedies by one person against another in respect of injuries of loss wrongfully caused' (Williams, 2006). If one person is found to be liable, then the outcome could, for example, be one of compensation offered to the injured.

*Criminal law* is a matter for society as a whole. In brief, these are sources of law that have a multitude of criminal conduct that exist in the criminal law. For the purpose of this chapter, the focus will be on those most applicable to Operating Department Practitioners. Statutory law are statutes that Acts of Parliament have brought into force after a series of procedural steps. Primary legislation is passed by Parliament; secondary legislation is regulations made by statutory instrument. This law sees the Crown on behalf of the State bring a case against a defendant. The outcome needs to show guilt beyond 'reasonable doubt' for a guilty verdict and if there is doubt the result will be not guilty. If the person is found guilty it can mean a prison sentence, community service or another punishment put in place. In Scotland there is a further possibility of an outcome and that is one of 'not proven'.

*Common law* generally describes the law that derived from judicial decision. English law is based on precedent where courts are obliged to follow previous decisions with relatively well-defined limits. This is why the use of particular cases has driven professional standards and guidelines; many will be discussed within the text.

### Stop and think

Before proceeding, list the laws you think impact on your individual practice and find out whether these are common law/criminal or civil?

## Legal statutes relating to practice

The statutes discussed include the Equality Act 2010; issues to do with consent, which includes the Mental Capacity Act 2005; the Children's Act 1989; confidentiality and the Data Protection Act 1998; the Human Tissue Act 2004 (2006 in Scotland); the Human Rights Act 1998; finishing with the Medicine Act 1968 and the Misuse of Drugs Act 1971. To ensure clarity there will be a brief description of each Act followed by its significance to the ODP.

*The Equality Act 2010* legally protects people from discrimination in the workplace and in wider society. It replaced previous anti-discrimination laws with a single Act, making the law easier to understand and strengthening protection in some situations. It sets out the different ways in which it is unlawful to treat someone. Before the Act came into force there were several pieces of legislation to cover discrimination, including the:

- Sex Discrimination Act 1975;
- Race Relations Act 1976;
- Disability Discrimination Act 1995.

It is against the law to discriminate against anyone because of: age; being or becoming a transsexual person; being married or in a civil partnership; being pregnant or having a child; race including colour, nationality, ethnic or national origin; religion, belief or lack of religion/belief; sex; and sexual orientation. These are called 'protected characteristics'.

Protection from discrimination is afforded to everyone in a variety of situations: for example, at work; in education; as a consumer; when using public services; when buying or renting property; and as a member or guest of a private club or association.

The ODP needs to be aware that they are treating patients in the NHS who are using a public service and therefore they should all be treated equally. In the independent sector, although not a public service, the patients are consumers of a service and have the same rights. As an employee you are also afforded the same rights not to be discriminated against under any of the protected characteristics.

As an individual we all have prejudices, whether conscious or unconscious. This could be termed as 'personal baggage' – and we can use the imagery of a rucksack on your back. The rucksack containing the prejudices needs to be removed while in your professional role. The 'personal baggage' will still be there but by consciously and physically separating it should not interfere with how you conduct yourself while in professional practice.

It is the role of all health professionals to challenge other professionals if they become aware of the discrimination or prejudicial behaviour. If you do have to challenge a colleague then your challenge should be timely and clearly state that you find the behaviour unacceptable. Remember that to fail to challenge the behaviour is effectively to condone the behaviour. If challenging unpleasant banter in the workplace, your challenge should be gentle but idle chit-chat, teasing and mocking can lead to covert discrimination and be offensive to colleagues. In most healthcare environments there will be local guidance on how to challenge this behaviour and where and to whom you should be taking your concerns. Discrimination is not acceptable in any work context. But by fostering a culture to challenge the behaviour or prejudices, it can avoid any escalation of workplace bullying.

## Consent

Consent has both a legal and ethical dimension. Valid consent must be obtained before starting treatment; physical investigation or providing personal care to a person. This reflects the right of patients to determine what happens to their own bodies, and is a fundamental part of good practice. While there is no English statute setting out the general principles of consent, case law ('common law') has established that touching a patient without valid consent may constitute the civil or criminal offence of battery. Furthermore, if ODPs (or any other healthcare staff) fail to obtain proper consent and the patient subsequently suffers harm as a result of treatment, a claim of negligence against the healthcare professional/s may be made.

Any healthcare professional (or other healthcare staff) who does not respect this may be liable under laws relating to assault and battery. The ODP would also be answerable to the regulator, the Health and Care Professions Council (HCPC), having breached their *Standards of Conduct, Performance and Ethics* (2012). Employing authorities could also be liable for the actions of their staff.

The ODP plays a significant role in checking to ensure that the correct consent has been sought. Where there is any concern this should be raised with the surgical and or anaesthetic team.

The *NHS Reference Guide to Consent for Treatment for Examination or Treatment* (2nd edn) (2009) provides details of the consent to physical interventions on patients from major surgery, administration or prescription of drugs to the assistance with dressing. The reference clearly sets clear guidance on who should seek consent, through to withdrawal and withholding of life-sustaining treatment. The guidance covers adults who do not have the capacity to consent, and also the gaining of consent on behalf of and by children. The ODP should be responsive to the differing approaches to consent and consider them in the context of the interventions performed as part of their role.

For consent to be valid, it must be voluntary and informed, and the person consenting must have the capacity to make the decision. These terms are explained as follows:

- Voluntary – the decision to consent or not to consent to treatment must be made by the person without any due pressure from family, friends or medical staff.
- Informed – the person must be given all the information about the treatment and what it involves. All the benefits and risks must be explained and nothing withheld. Alternative treatments should also be discussed. This is usually done by a medical practitioner but not necessarily, as it should be conducted by whoever is doing the intervention.

The capacity of the person to understand the information given to them is paramount for them to make an informed decision and to give consent. If the person refuses treatment then their decision should be respected at whatever stage of process they are at. This is still true even if their decision would result in their death, or the death of their unborn child.

Consent can be given verbally, non-verbally or in writing. Familiarity with the employing authorities' consent forms is essential; however, they are not a legal requirement but serve to provide evidence of consent but the completion of a consent form is irrelevant if the consent is not voluntary or informed. It is essential to be familiar with your employing authorities' local policy regarding consent. This is important, as the policy will tie in with the indemnity offered to staff as part of their employment. Consent should be obtained in advance allowing the patient sufficient time to ask questions and this ideally should be supported with a written information sheet setting out the procedure.

## Unable to give consent

Patients who lack capacity should not be denied necessary treatment simply because they are unable to give consent. The Mental Capacity Act (2005) formalizes the area assessing whether the patient is mentally capable of making the decision, and the Mental Health Acts (1983 and amended in 2007) describe the very limited circumstances when a patient can be forced to be hospitalized for assessment and/or treatment against their wishes. The Act also applies where decisions have to be made on behalf of persons lacking capacity. The decision to act should always be with regard to the patient's personal health and wellbeing.

There are procedural circumstances where if someone is unable to give consent, these decision need to be referred to the Court of Protection. Situations that should always be referred to the courts include:

- sterilization for contraceptive purposes;
- donation of regenerative tissue, such as bone marrow;
- withdrawal of nutrition and hydration from a person who is in a persistent vegetative state;
- where there is serious concern about the person's capacity or best interests.

Where a person lacks capacity to give consent, it is essential that the ODP is aware of the legal statute with regard to dealing with these patients.

## Mental Capacity Act 2005

### 'Best interest' under the Mental Capacity Act 2005

The Mental Capacity Act 2005 is complex but many sources of guidance have been developed. Dr Theresa Joyce authored a document on behalf of the British Psychological Society, which was published by the Department of Health (DH) in 2007, *Best Interest, Guidance on Determining the Best Interest of Adults Who Lack Capacity to Make a Decision (or Decisions) for Themselves (England and Wales) December 2007*. This document provides clear information and support to the multidisciplinary team who may be participating in decisions on behalf of adults who lack the capacity to do so for themselves. Although the guidance is not specifically aimed at the perioperative environment, it has relevance to the ODP regarding an understanding of the legal issues involved and the patients where they may be participating in their care.

In brief, the guidance raises awareness of the different ways in which people can make decisions on behalf of those who lack capacity and the relevance to the Mental Capacity Act 2005. It aims to help practitioners who work with individuals that lack capacity and who are required to make judgements about best interest to ensure that they weigh up all the relevant factors in making those decisions. A patient coming to theatre who may have a long-term condition, such as Alzheimer's disease, will have gone through a process to establish that the surgery to be performed has been done in the 'best interest' of the patient. The ODP will need to be aware that the records clearly state that:

the grounds on which they have reached this decision, the treatment which will be undertaken, and how this treatment will be in the patient's best interests. It is good practice – but not a legal requirement – to contact and seek the approval of relatives or others significant to the patient, but failure to do so should not compromise care in an emergency.

(Association of Anaethetists of Great Britain and Ireland (AAGBI), 2006: 9)

It is therefore important that the ODP is aware of the considerations that have to be part of the 'best interest' decision.

The Act defines what 'lacking capacity' means. So where a person has made their wishes known in an advance decision (or otherwise known as advance directives (AD)) or as an end of life statement, it helps clinicians in treatment decisions. The advance decision is legally binding in England and Wales, although the actual patient has the right to override what is written in the statement or whatever their legal representative says. In Scotland and Northern Ireland the matter is covered by common law as opposed to legislation. It will be upheld if the intentions are clear and the adult does not lack capacity.

A reference document that ODPs may find useful, although not specifically focused on the perioperative area, is the National Council for Palliative Care and the National End of Life Care Programme, *Advance Decision to Refuse Treatment – A Guide for Health and Social Care Professionals* (January 2013). Its focus is on the health and social care, but it has a good insight into approaches for making decisions for others. Areas where this could impact on the ODP in practice are:

- the use of intravenous fluids and parenteral nutrition;
- the use of cardiopulmonary resuscitation;
- the use of life-saving treatment (whether existing or yet to be developed) in specific illnesses where capacity or consent may be impaired; for example, brain damage, perhaps from stroke, head injury or dementia;
- specific procedures such as blood transfusion for a patient who does not consent to this treatment; for example, a patient who is a Jehovah's Witness.

In brief, the document explains the process on how decisions should be made:

- *Advance decisions* are about refusing treatment that is legally binding providing they meet certain conditions. If these conditions are met, then they should be followed, even if they do not appear to be in the best interests of the person who now lacks capacity.

- *Substituted judgement decisions* are included where the known views or wishes of the person when they had capacity have to be considered.
- Best interests' decisions weighs up a range of factors (including the wishes or preferences of the person, and the views of their families and carers) and these are decided on what is, on balance, the best for the person both now and in the future.

### Case law

It may be useful to look at some case law on the right to refuse treatment. The following two cases, found in Kennedy and Grubb (2000), are well known. The first was cited in the second case as a point of precedence.

*Re C (Adult, refusal of treatment)* [1994] 1 All ER 819
The right of a competent adult to refuse medical treatment. The principle that mental illness does not automatically call a patient's capacity into question

Re C had paranoid schizophrenia and was detained in Broadmoor secure hospital. He developed gangrene in his leg but refused to agree to an amputation, which doctors considered was necessary to save his life. The Court upheld C's decision.

- The fact that a person has a mental illness does not automatically mean they lack capacity to make a decision about medical treatment.
- Patients who have capacity (i.e. who can understand, believe, retain and weigh the necessary information) can make their own decisions to refuse treatment, even if those decisions appear irrational to the doctor or may place the patient's health or their life at risk.

*Re MB (Adult, medical treatment)* [1997] 38 BMLR 175 CA
Capacity to refuse treatment

MB needed a caesarean section, but panicked and withdrew consent at the last moment because of her needle phobia. The hospital obtained a judicial declaration that it would be lawful to carry out the procedure, a decision that MB appealed against. However, she subsequently agreed to the induction of anaesthesia and her baby was born by caesarean section.

The Court of Appeal upheld the judges' view that MB had not, at the time, been competent to refuse treatment, taking the view that her fear and panic had impaired her capacity to take in the information she was given about her condition and the proposed treatment. In assessing the case the judges reaffirmed the test of capacity set out in the Re C judgment.

- An individual's capacity to make particular decisions may fluctuate or be temporarily affected by factors such as pain, fear, confusion or the effects of medication.
- Assessment of capacity must be timely and decision-specific.

The two cases demonstrate the rights of the patients and the difficulty for medical staff when trying to assess the capacity of the patient to make an informed decision.

## Children's Act 1989

The Children's Act 1989 Act covers all aspects of children's services, including education, welfare and health. The most significant aspect of this act for ODPs is around the rights of the child in determining their care, especially regarding consent and treating children and their families with safeguarding and respect. Due to the complexity of the Act and to provide direction, implementation documents under the National Service Framework (NSF) were produced. *Getting the Right Start: Nation Service Framework for Children* (DH, 2003a) set out a 10-year plan outlining targets within health and social care to improve services for children. The NSF for Children, 'Standard for hospital services', 2003 set out some key aspects that relate and impact on the role of the ODP. For example the NSF states that 'where care is provided for children there must be staff trained in life support' (NSF, 2003: 22). Whereas basic life support is usually sufficient in most areas within the surgical recovery area and day case facilities, there should be at least one person with a Paediatric Advanced Life Support (PALS) qualification. This also includes the availability of drugs and equipment to stabilize a critically ill child. All staff who work with children also need to ensure they are 'trained, updated, supported and supervized in safeguarding children and promoting of their well being' (DH, 2003a: 23). ODPs should be aware of their professional accountability in relation to having the appropriate knowledge and skills when working with children.

**Stop and think**

Think of the facilities you have in your department in relation to children. What training have practitioners undertaken? How would you like to improve services to children who come to your operating theatre?

### Children and consent

Following a case in 1982 where a mother, named Victoria Gillick, took her local health authority (West Norfolk and Wisbech Area Health Authority) and the DH and Social Security (DHSS) to court in an attempt to stop doctors from giving contraceptive advice or treatment to under 16-year-olds without parental consent.

*Gillick* v. *West Norfolk and Wisbech AHA* [1986] AC 112
Children and young people's competence to consent to treatment

Mrs Gillick challenged the lawfulness of DH guidance that doctors could provide contraceptive advice and treatment to girls under the age of 16 without parental consent or knowledge in some circumstances.

The House of Lords upheld that a doctor could give contraceptive advice and treatment to a young person under the age of 16 if:

- she had sufficient maturity and intelligence to understand the nature and implications of the proposed treatment;
- she could not be persuaded to tell her parents or to allow her doctor to tell them;
- she was very likely to begin or continue having sexual intercourse with or without contraceptive treatment;
- her physical or mental health were likely to suffer unless she received the advice or treatment;
- the advice or treatment was in the young person's best interests.

Although this case was about contraceptive advice, it has been used as the point in law regarding the capability of children under 16 being able to consent to treatment. Kennedy notes Lord Scarman's comments in his judgment of the Gillick case in the House of Lords (1985) that are often referred to as the test of 'Gillick competency': the child or young person should be able to understand the nature of the advice while have sufficient maturity to comprehend what is involved. The Fraser guidelines refer to the guidelines set out by Lord Fraser in his judgment of the Gillick case in the House of Lords (1985).

'Fraser guidelines' and 'Gillick competence' are terms that are often used and are interchangeable as the premise of both is about the right of the child, who has sufficient understanding, to decide on their treatment or procedure. Awareness of the child's rights, in any given situation in the perioperative environment, is paramount particularly in their right to refuse treatment. This can give rise to anxiety and frustration to those present, to the parent/carers who will naturally feel responsible. The ODP will need to ensure that they are supportive to both the child and the parents/guardians and use their skill of empathic communication to ensure the right outcome is achieved. The child's right to refuse does depend on having sufficient competence and understanding and it is the role of the ODP and other health professionals to listen, support and respect their decision.

### Points of law on negligence

Negligence occurs when there is a failure in the duty of care provided and the patient incurs an injury or some form of damage. A breach in the duty of care was cited in a case of *Bolam* v. *Friern Hospital Management Committee* [1957] 1 W.L.R. 583, 587. The case is about a man who had electro convulsive therapy and was not given a muscle relaxant or provided with adequate restraint, which resulted in him sustaining serious injuries and fractures. The case gave rise to the term widely used now as the 'Bolam test'. The judge stated that the skill used could not be judged against that of the ordinary man but against that of one with specialist skill; therefore, a doctor is not negligent if he acts in accordance accepted by a responsible body of fellow medical men.

This benchmark would be true for ODPs using the same measure and standard of practice. Therefore, the judgment of negligence would be in accordance to what a reasonable body of fellow ODPs skilled in that practice would feel is appropriate.

### Stop and think

How often in practice do you speak with colleagues about the way you are working and whether the way you are practising is of an agreed standard? Take one aspect of your daily routine and explore this with others to gain an understanding of current practice.

## Confidentiality

Patient confidentiality is bound by professional practice and all ODPs are bound by the law of the Data Protection Act 1998, NHS Codes of Practice on Confidentiality, and HCPC Standards of Proficiency 2014, HCPC Standards of Conduct Performance and Ethics 2012 and contracts of employment. It is encompassed in common law and statute, as well as protecting human rights as seen in the European Convention of Human Rights.

Confidentiality is governed by the Data Protection Act 1998 and it clearly states that people have a right to expect information to only be used in relation to the reason it was given. They also have a right to control access to their own personal health information, which means ODPs cannot discuss matters relating to patients outside the clinical setting where they could potentially not be overheard, nor leave records unattended where they may be read by others. Looking through patients' notes should also be on a 'need to know' basis to inform you and others of any condition relevant to their care. Although the patient has a legal right to gain access to their health records, it is inappropriate to do so in the perioperative environment. All verbal requests should be directed towards the employing authority's procedure for gaining access to health records.

Confidentiality forms an important part of the trust between health professionals and patients. The patient has a right to privacy, and when they confide in the health professional with their personal details, they expect that the information will not be disclosed unless required to help with their treatment. The NHS Code of Practice (2003), governed by the Data Protection Act 1998, states that patients' health information and their interests must be protected through a number of measures:

- procedures to ensure that all staff, contractors and volunteers are at all times fully aware of their responsibilities regarding confidentiality;
- recording patient information accurately and consistently;
- keeping patient information private;
- keeping patient information physically secure;
- disclosing and using information with appropriate care.

The ODP needs to be aware of discussing cases in public areas and particularly in operating theatre corridors, movement and transfer between anaesthetic, surgical and post-anaesthetic areas, changing rooms and rest areas. These areas are predominately frequented by other healthcare staff, and, at times, the general public. Information sharing is acceptable if seeking advice, sharing an experience or knowledge, but a patient's identity should not be disclosed. Be aware that key details can easily lead to a person's identity becoming evident, and gossiping is never acceptable. Students and practitioners doing further study should be aware of the pitfalls of breaching confidentiality when writing and sharing experiences and therefore students should ensure they are familiar with their university confidentiality guidelines.

It is the practitioner's responsibility to keep patient's details secure. This means not leaving patient details and files open on a computer screen and following the correct procedure for logging out. Medical notes and paper files should never be left unattended or in an easily accessible area. Vigilance between the team is essential and making others aware of any potential breach is good practice.

There are exemptions to maintaining confidentiality and these are clearly laid out in criteria where breaching confidentiality is justified. The criteria are set out in a DH document, *Confidentiality: NHS Code of Practice. Supplementary Guidance Public Interest* (2010). The document expands the principles in the original DH key guidance on *Confidentiality: NHS Code of Practice* (2003b) and is aimed at supporting staff in making difficult decisions about when disclosures of confidential information may be justified in the public interest.

Examples of where public interest can be a defence include:

- Reporting to the Driver & Vehicle Licensing Centre a patient who rejects medical advice not to drive (although health professionals should inform the patient of their intention to report it);
- Breaching the confidentiality of a patient who refuses to inform his or her sexual partner of a serious sexually transmissible infection;
- Releasing relevant confidential information to social services where there is a potential risk of significant harm to a child.

(DH, *Confidentiality: NHS Code of Practice*, 2010: 9)

## Whistle blowing in the NHS – The Public Interest Disclosure Act 1998

The Public Interest Disclosure Act became law in 1999 and was further supported by a Health Service Circular HSC 1999/198 that set out the rationale for all NHS Trusts and Health Authorities to develop a whistle-blowing policy. The circular gave protection to employees who wanted to make a protected disclosure of information regarding matters relating to their employment. The protection included the person not being dismissed or penalized by their employers as a result of the disclosure. The whistle-blowing provisions make the confidentiality clauses unenforceable in agreements between workers and employers.

The employee who is intending to use the whistle-blowing provision would need to ensure that the disclosure met with one or more of the following areas:

- that a criminal offence has been committed, is being committed or is likely to be committed;
- that a person has failed, is failing or is likely to fail to comply with any legal obligation to which he is subject;
- that a miscarriage of justice has occurred, is occurring or is likely to occur;
- that the health or safety of any individual has been, is being or is likely to be endangered;
- that the environment has been, is being or is likely to be damaged, or that information tending to show any matter falling within any one of the preceding paragraphs has been, or is likely to be deliberately concealed.

The circumstances in which you may make disclosures vary depending on the recipient. You should make the disclosure in accordance with your employer's whistle-blowing policy. Such policies should identify the person that you should speak to if you have concerns about taking it to your employer.

The ODP has a responsibility to act to protect the public and if you witness and/or have concerns about malpractice in your workplace the Act will protect 'whistle blowers' against victimization or dismissal, provided they have behaved responsibly in dealing with their concerns.

## Raising and escalating concerns

At times, concerns may arise where the ODP does not wish to follow the formal whistle-blowing policy. In this situation the regulator (HCPC) has set out some guiding principles in raising and escalating concerns regarding another professional's fitness to practice. The ODP has a duty to act upon concerns as set out in standard 1 of the Standards of Conduct, Performance and Ethics, which requires you to 'act in the best interests of your service users' (HCPC, 2012: 8).

This should be brought to the attention of your manager in the first place or if this is not appropriate to a senior manager in the organization. The matter may be able to be addressed internally; however, if for any reason this is not addressed in a timely manner, then you should take this further up the organization or to the professional regulatory body.

### Conscientious objection to participation in treatment

There may be reasons for an ODP to raise a conscientious objection to participate in treatment of a patient. In law there are two areas where the right to refuse to participate in the treatment is accepted. Article 4(2) of the Abortion Act 1967 (Scotland, England and Wales): the right to refuse to have direct involvement in abortion procedures and Article 38(2) of the Human and Fertilisation and Embryology Act (2008): the right to refuse to participate in technological procedures to achieve conception and pregnancy. Therefore, if there are any legal proceedings the burden of proof of conscientious objection will be with the person claiming to rely on it.

The Abortion Act 1967 does however place a caveat within subsection (1) 'there is nothing that shall affect any duty to participate in treatment which is necessary to save the life or to prevent grave permanent injury to the physical or mental health of a pregnant woman' (Abortion Act, page. 3, section 4). This means that in the case of an emergency you have a duty to participate and not omit care required and act in the best interest of the patient. Any ODP who wishes to make it known that they are a conscientious objector should speak with a senior member of staff, and following this up in writing stating that they do not wish to participate in the practice. The practitioner should do this as soon as possible and in advance. It would be unacceptable to do so once the patient has presented as it may cause staffing and care delivery issues that could cause harm to the patient.

**Stop and think**

As an ODP in charge of a list, how would you handle this situation?

Staffing was short due to sickness. A health professional had been assigned to your operating list at short notice by a senior member of staff. It was not until they arrived that they realized the list they had been asked to work on was a very busy termination of pregnancies list. The health professional informed you they would not participate in the list as they were a conscientious objector, and had put this in writing some time ago.

### Human Tissue Act 2004 (2006 in Scotland)

The removal of products, specimens' and samples is common practice within the operating theatre and therefore the Human Tissue Act is relevant to the activities of the ODP. The Act regulates how the removal, storage and use of human tissue from either the living or the dead is organized and controlled. This includes any organs or residual tissue following clinical and diagnostic procedures. The Human Tissue Act (2004) makes consent a legal requirement for the removal, storage and use of human tissue or organs and sets out whose consent is needed in which circumstances. The Human Tissue Authority (HTA) is the licensing body responsible for approving the transplantation of organs from living donors, including bone marrow and peripheral blood stem cells from adults who lack the capacity to consent and children who lack the competence to consent. The HTA also license activity regarding stem cells and how they are removed, stored and processed. Since 2008, anybody collecting cord blood needs to be doing so under the licence of the HTA. It covers the collection, the quality of the samples and how they are stored; the consent of the mother and the lawful use of the sample. The ODP may see this activity following caesarean section where it is the wishes of the parents.

### What is the Human Rights Act?

The Human Rights Act 1998 is a law that has as its core values fairness, respect, equality and dignity. It came into force in the UK in October 2000 and included the rights enshrined in the European Convention on Human Rights. Article 2 is significant to the role of the ODP as it deals with the right to life, issues such as do not resuscitate orders, refusal of life saving medical treatment, advanced directives and death through negligence. Although this has the most significance the other main articles that are also relevant in medical law are: Article 2 (protection of the right to life), Article 3 (prohibition of torture and inhuman or degrading treatment or punishment), Article 5 (the right to liberty and security), Article 8 (the right to respect for private and family life), Article 9 (freedom of thought, conscience and religion), Article 12 (the right to marry and found a family) and Article 14 (prohibition of discrimination in the enjoyment of Convention rights).

Within healthcare, the Human Rights Act is all about balancing different people's rights and often:

rights appear to conflict with each other, judgements have to be made about priorities or boundaries. There are many instances in NHS organizations where rights have to be balanced to protect the safety or rights of others, or in the interests of good order. For example, ensuring that staff is protected from violent or abusive patients while also having regard to the interests of the patient.

(DH and BIHR, 2008)

## Drug legislation

The handling of drugs is very much a part of the ODP's role. Therefore knowledge and understanding of the legislation is paramount as ignorance is no defence in the eyes of the law. Changes occur over time to the regulation and legislation and it is essential that the ODP remains current by using the reference points presented.

### Medicines Act 1968

The Medicines Act 1968 is the guiding legislation controlling the manufacturing and distribution of medicinal products. It is often referred to as primary legislation and cross-referred to when amendments or further regulations are developed or changed. The significance of the Act is that it sets out the legal status of drugs and their classification regarding penalties.

Each medicinal product is given a legal status and this correlates to how the medicines can be supplied.

- on a prescription (referred to as prescription only medicines (POMs));
- in a pharmacy without prescription, under the supervision of a pharmacist (P);
- on general sale (GSL) and can be sold in general retail outlets without the supervision of a pharmacist.

*Note:* Prescriptions can be issued by doctors, dentists, regulated professional independent prescribers, pharmacist independent prescribers and supplementary prescribers.

The regulation of medicines is the responsibility of the Medicines and Healthcare Products Regulatory Agency (MHRA), who are also responsible for medical devices and equipment used in healthcare, and the investigation of harmful incidents. The MHRA also have responsibility for blood and blood products, working with UK blood services, healthcare providers, and other relevant organizations to improve blood quality and safety. They provide excellent online information for theatre practitioners such as guidance, safety alerts and interactive educational material. The Medicines Act gives the overarching framework for drug legislation but the most familiar piece of legislation to ODPs will be the Misuse of Drugs Act 1971 governing controlled drugs.

### Misuse of Drugs Act 1971

The Misuse of Drugs Act 1971 is divided into regulations that have as part of this the classification related to the misuse of drugs, the scheduling of drugs and the safe custody. The UK misuse classification of drugs is set out into three classes. Class A, B and C that relate to the risk of harm the drug poses to individuals or to society by its misuse. Class A drugs pose a very high risk of harm and these are heroin, cocaine, methadone, ecstasy, LSD and magic mushrooms. Class B drugs include amphetamines, barbiturates, codeine, cannabis and synthetic cannabis. Class C drugs include benzodiazepines (tranquillizers) GHB, anabolic steroids, GBL and benzylpiperazines. The classification and the misuse are reflected in the period of sentencing and fines incurred. These vary depending on whether in possession or whether there is intent to sell. This will also depend on the amount of drugs involved, the previous criminal record and the circumstances of the offences.

The scheduling of drugs is controlled by the Misuse of Drugs Regulations 2001 that divides drugs into five schedules, and these correspond to their therapeutic, usefulness and misuse potential. A number of changes affecting the prescribing, record keeping and destruction of controlled drugs have been introduced as a result of amendments to the Misuse of Drugs Regulations 2001. In 2006 amendments were made to the regulations in response to safe management of medicine; and in 2007 an amendment was made giving the authority to ODPs to possess and supply controlled drugs, prior to this it only states that a senior registered nurse could do this (Home Office circular 027/2007).

The schedules relate to the recording, administration and disposal of a drug. The ODP will be accountable for keeping clear, timely and correct records of drugs they supply to a medical practitioner or independent prescriber. The drugs mentioned under the following schedules are the ones the ODP will have most exposure to within the operating theatre and related areas.

- Schedule 1 drugs have no recognizable medical use – such as raw opium and hallucinogens.
- Schedule 2 is pharmaceutical opiates used during and post-anaesthesia. A register must be kept for Schedule 2 CDs and this register must comply with the relevant regulations.
- Schedule 3 contain barbiturates.
- Schedule 4 contain benzodiazepines.
- Schedule 5 contains drugs found in schedule 2 but is of a lesser concentration such as cocaine paste.

In the event that an ODP has to dispose of a residual amount of drug left in a syringe following a case they must do so in accordance with their employing authority. There is guidance from the Royal Pharmaceutical Society of Great Britain (RPSGB, 2007) on the destruction of controlled drugs, which states that all drugs must be destroyed in a manner that is appropriate and safe.

Any medicines should be disposed of in relevant waste containers that are then sent for incineration and should not be disposed of in the sewerage system. All CDs in Schedule 2, 3 and 4 (part I) can be placed into waste containers only after the controlled drug has been rendered irretrievable (i.e. by denaturing). Local policy needs to be followed.

ODPs can administer any prescribed drug under schedules 2, 3 and 4 or any drug under the directions of a medical practitioner. Many employing authorities have intravenous drug administration training programmes that staff have to undertake to be covered by the local policy. All ODPs should gain access to these to ensure that they comply with the vicarious liability of the employing authority.

As many ODPs are in regular contact with drugs as part of their role, it is paramount that they remain current and up to date in the changes to any regulations. It is important to recognize that a medicine or device may hold a product licence, but should there be any change, such as a strength of a drug or the change of use for a piece of equipment, the responsibility for the quality of its use will lie with a healthcare professional, whether this is an ODP or medical practitioner.

## Conclusion

The legislation discussed in this chapter represents the key areas that impact on the ODP's working practice. The role of the ODP has changed and developed over the years and with this has come a greater responsibility and accountability to understand the areas of the law that are within their scope of practice. Many of these will be translated into policies and procedures of your employing authority. The overview of the law given in this chapter directs the practitioner to the legal fundamentals related to their role. It will require the practitioner to remain updated on any changes that affect their way of working. Wider reading will be necessary and invaluable within your own area of practice, particularly if in an advanced role.

## Key points

- ODPs understanding of legal terms and how they impact on their practice.
- Why consent and confidentiality are so key to the rights of the patients and the responsibility and accountability of the ODP.
- Gain a clear understanding of the drug legislation and that it is the responsibility of the ODP to remain up to date and current on any changes.

## References and further reading

Association of Anaesthetists for Great Britain and Ireland (AAGBI) (2006) *Consent for Anaesthesia* (2nd edn). London: AAGBI.

*Bolam* v. *Friern Hospital Management Committee* [1957] 1 W.L.R. 583, 587.

Children's Act 1989. Available online at www.legislation.gov.uk search children act 1989

Department of Health (DH) (2003a) *Getting the Right Start: National Service Framework for Children. Standard for Hospital Services*. London: DH. Available online at https://www.gov.uk/government/publications/national-service-framework-children-young-people-and-maternity-services

Department of Health (DH) (2003b) *Confidentiality – NHS Code of Practice*. London: DH. Available online at https://www.gov.uk/government/publications/confidentiality-nhs-code-of-practice (accessed 30 August 2013).

Department of Health (DH) (2009) *Reference Guide to Consent for Examination or Treatment* (2nd edn). London: DH. Available online at https://www.gov.uk/government/publications/reference-guide-to-consent-for-examination-or-treatment-second-edition (accessed January 2013).

Department of Health (DH) (2010) *Confidentiality – NHS Code of Practice* (updated from 2003b). DH: London. Available online at https://www.gov.uk/government/publications/confidentiality-nhs-code-of-practice (accessed 30 August 2013).

Department of Health (DH) (2010) *Confidentiality: NHS Code of Practice – Supplementary Guidance Public Interest*. London: DH.

Department of Health (DH) and British Institute of Human Rights (BIHR) (2008) *Human Rights in Healthcare: A Framework for Local Action* (2nd edn). London: DH. Available online at www.equalityhumanrights.com (accessed 20 July 2012).

Equality Act (2010) *Guidance*. Available online at www.gov.uk/equality-act-2010-guidance (accessed March 2013).

*Gillick* v. *West Norfolk and Wisbech Area Health Authority* [1985] AC 112 (HL).

Health and Care Professions Council (HCPC) (2012) *Standards of Conduct, Performance and Ethics for ODPs*. London: HCPC.

Home Office Circular (027/2007) Available online at www.gov.uk/government/publications/misuse-of-drugs-and-misuse-of-drugs-safe-custody-amendment-regulations-2007 (accessed 10 March 2013).

Human Rights Act 1998. Available online at www.legislation.gov.uk

Human Tissues Act (2004) (Scotland 2006). Available online at www.legislation.gov.uk

Joyce, T. (2007) British Psychological Society *Best Interest, Guidance on Determining the Best Interest of Adults who Lack Capacity to Make a Decision (or Decisions) for Themselves (England And Wales)*. London: DH.

Kennedy, I. and Grubb, A. (2000) *Medical Law* (3rd edn). London: Butterworth.

Medicine Act 1968 Available online at http://www.legislation.gov.uk/ukpga/1968/67 (accessed 15 August 2013).

Medicines and Healthcare Products Regulatory Agency (MHRA). Available online at www.mhra.gov.uk (accessed 12 August 2013).

Mental Capacity Act 2005. Available online at www.legislation.gov.uk

Misuse of Drugs Regulation 2001. Available online at www.legislation.gov.uk

National Council for Palliative Care and the National End of Life Care Programme (2013) *Advance Decision to Refuse Treatment: A Guide for Health and Social Care Professionals. End of Life Care Programme.* Available at http://www.endoflifecare.nhs.uk/search-resources/resources-search/publications/imported-publications/advance-decisions-to-refuse-treatment.aspx (accessed 30 May 2013).

Public Interest Disclosure Act 1998. Available online at www.legislation.gov.uk

Public Interest Disclosure Act 1998. *Whistleblowing in the NHS Health*, Service Circular HSC 1999/198. Available online at www.dh.gov.uk

Royal Pharmaceutical Society for Great Britain (RPSGB) (2007) *Guidance for Pharmacists on the Safe Destruction of Controlled Drugs: England, Scotland and Wales.* London: RPSGB.

The Abortion Act 1967. Available online at www.legislation.gov.uk

The Misuse of Drugs and Misuse of Drugs (safe custody) (amendment) Regulation 2007. Available online at www.legislation.gov.uk

Williams, G. (2006) *Learning the Law* (13th edn). London: Sweet and Maxwell.

# 7 Ethics for the Operating Department Practitioner

## *Helen Booth*

**Key topics**

- Why ethics is relevant to Operating Department Practitioners (ODPs)

- How ethical theories impact on ODP practice

- Understanding guiding principles to standards of behaviour

- How values play a part in working practice

- Framework of questions to support ethical problems and decision making

## Introduction

The professionalization of operating department practice, and the changes in healthcare over recent years has meant that practitioners face increasingly complex situations and difficult decisions in practice. This chapter explores the underpinning ethical principles that can shape and guide the ODP in making these decisions.

The key areas that are explored are the principles and theories of ethics, and how they guide standards of behaviour in practice. It also considers how ODPs engage with other health professionals to ensure a collective approach to the care of the patient. The professional regulatory standards and guidelines are not discussed in detail as, although they act as a useful reference point, they are founded on good professional experience and influenced by legal statute.

## Why is ethics relevant to ODPs?

Ethics refers to standards of behaviour that tell us how human beings ought to act in many situations, especially within professional roles. As part of their professional role, the ODP will inevitably have to consider the ethical implications of care and changing care. Many would consider ethics as mere 'common sense', but common sense is usually founded upon experience and personal beliefs. However, beliefs and norms are not universal. It is therefore important to make a distinction between what are personal beliefs, which may or may not comply with others, and common sense, which are accepted as a standard by most reasonable people most of the time. When entering a profession and meeting ethics in professional life for the first time you will often hear phrases such as 'isn't that obvious?', and 'isn't that just common sense?'. This is understandable, but it is important to remember that this impression is based on the learned behaviour from a particular individual's culture, social experience and peers. This is obviously of value and forms the basis of most ethical frameworks. However, this approach is not sufficient or structured enough when dealing with the wide complexity within healthcare, and the daily complexities of dealing with patients and colleagues within the perioperative environment. Ethics is an integral part of professional life and therefore require the practitioner to develop a deeper understanding of the subject area.

The term 'ethics' is a principle that guides human behaviour, and morals are associated with those that guide social behaviour. Before exploring these terms in further detail, it is useful to clarify what ethics is not:

- Ethics is not just about feelings (though feelings do often play a part in ethical choices).
- Ethics is not about religion or following cultural norms as ethical principles are equally applicable to all.
- Ethics is not about following the law, although there are references to standards of behaviour.
- Ethics is not a science, as it cannot always be quantified and measured, although ethics within science is important, particularly within the context of research.

This shows some of the complexity surrounding professional ethics, and poses questions for an ODP's practice and decision making.

The theories and principles of ethics provide a framework for debate, discussion, disagreement and understanding. There are a number of useful theories explained in the following section that may be useful to your understanding of these debates. Although they may not seem immediately relevant to everyday situations, they will help with difficult decision making in practice. ODPs now practice in such varied healthcare settings that it is impossible to address all ethical problems and dilemmas that you might be faced with. However, a framework of questions has been developed in this chapter to use as an aid for exploring ethical dilemmas in practice.

In healthcare, ethical standards are well founded in codes and guidance. They prescribe what a practitioner should or should not do, usually in the terms of rights, obligations, benefits to the patients and the upholding of specific virtues. The basis underpinning ethical standards and the relevant philosophers, and how they relate to the ODP, are discussed.

## Ethical theories

The following section examines the theories relevant to the practice of the ODP with some examples of how these are translated to practical matters. The theories covered are utilitarianism, consequentialism, duty-based ethics and the 'four principle' approach that has guided the professional ethical standards over the last 30 years. There are many more ethical approaches but none that are as well known for their application to practical issues and the values they represent.

### Utilitarianism

The major philosophers who developed the utilitarian approach were Jeremy Bentham (1748–1832) and John Stuart Mill (1806–1873). Mill (1867) describes the theory as being based upon producing the greatest happiness for the greater number of people. Happiness is equated to good.

Utilitarianism considers an action as morally right if its outcome or consequences are good for the greatest number in society. The theory tends to disregard individual rights and considers the well-being of the greatest number to be the most important factor. In the healthcare context, utilitarianism becomes evident in discussions about the allocation of resources. With only a finite amount of money to spend on healthcare, decisions on where and how it should be spent is a challenge. On a micro level the ODP will be aware of the day-to-day resource allocation of equipment and disposables. However, the macro-level decisions of a healthcare organization are usually utilitarian where there is the greatest need within a demographic area. The utilitarian approach would be to advocate doing whatever brought the greatest good and happiness to the greatest amount of people. A good example of this can be seen in the UK vaccination programmes. The vaccination programme afforded by the UK has shown proven benefits in eradicating many childhood diseases. However, due to an unreliable research paper in 1998 regarding the measles, mumps and rubella (MMR) vaccine, there has been a recorded rise in measles that has not been seen for decades. In this example it clearly shows the benefits of a utilitarian approach where having a vaccination programme provides the greatest benefits to the greater number of people.

### Consequentialism

Consequentialism (or teleology as it is sometimes called) is concerned with the consequences or outcomes of an action rather than the deed itself. This theory has a premise of the utilitarian approach and related to the greater good on the outcome or consequences of the act. However, it does have limitations as it can endorse acts that would be contrary to the rights of the individual. The action taken is morally correct as long as the consequences are beneficial. For example, if an ODP felt they needed to breach confidentiality on a matter regarding the patient, the practitioner would need to weigh up the consequences of the action. The ODP may think that the breach has perceived benefits to others but to the individual patient it could be viewed as a betrayal of trust. Consequences in any given situation are often difficult to predict. The action may have had good intentions and have a high probability of there being a good result. But, if something was to happen and the consequences had a bad outcome then the action of the ODP is morally wrong. In many situations that involve a number of people and options, it becomes more difficult to establish which action would produce the best outcome/consequence.

### Duty based/deontology

The best-known advocate for duty-based ethics was Immanuel Kant who founded this theory based on the correctness of an action regardless of the harm or benefits it may produce. Kant (1964) believed that it was feasible to develop a consistent moral system by using reason. The belief is that there are particular duties that must be upheld at any cost – an unconditional moral law could be applied to all rational beings. Kant called this a 'categorical imperative', and suggested three ways in which this could be carried out:

- Act in such a way that your actions can and ought to be universal.
- Treat people as ends in themselves and never solely as the means to an end.
- Act in such a way as you would have someone act towards you.

So, duty ethics would not say that you can justify an action just because it produces a good outcome. The emphasis is on valuing the human being and giving equal respect to all.

Kant's theory of categorical imperative became the foundation underpinning the 'principle' approach to ethics that lies in the 'respect for persons'. It is an arguable one that spans all aspects of life whether in health or other. It is only right that any individual is worthy of respect, whether we like them or not. It is the foundation on how we should treat others. It could be potentially the only over-arching principle and value needed for all professionals in a given work situation and relates to the value afforded to both our patients and colleagues.

### Stop and think

Look at this scenario and discuss the ethical aspects in relation to consequential and duty ethics theories.

Imagine that an ODP attends to someone in the street who was having a cardiac arrest and resuscitated them successfully. Due to unforeseen circumstances while undertaking the resuscitation, the ODP cracked several ribs and bruised the person's chest badly, which resulted in some long-term problems for the person's recovery. Using the two ethical approaches, discuss and debate this brief scenario to enable you to create a deeper understanding within the professional context.

### Principles theory

This approach has become the most popular theory in healthcare ethics and the principles provide useful insights to problem solving. It is based on a set of principles developed by Beauchamp and Childress in the early 1980s in their 2001 book entitled *Principles of Biomedical Ethics*. They state that the 'four cluster of principles' do not constitute a general moral theory. They provide only a framework for identifying and reflecting on moral problems (Beauchamp and Childress, 2001: 15).

A principle is an essential norm in a system of thought or belief, forming a basis of moral reasoning in that system. The 'four principles' are written in a broad term so that they have a wider scope and can be applied to all people in any situation. However, principle-based theories usually infer ethical reasoning and decision making as a rational process of applying principles.

The 'four principles' identified by Beauchamp and Childress are autonomy, beneficence, nonmaleficence and justice. These are briefly explored as follows:

1. Autonomy – this principle is a primary consideration for patient-centred care. It promotes the ability of the person to be independent and self-determining and to make a reasoned choice on the basis of information. It is a highly significant principle in healthcare as it implies that the patient has the right not to be constrained, coerced or impeded in any way. It requires respect for the person and for the ODP to promote and not obstruct their patients' autonomy. However, where this may not be possible, the ODP should follow the principle of beneficence.
2. Beneficence – this principle considers the balance of treatment against the risks and costs to the patients. Therefore the ODP should always act in a way that benefits the patient, although it may be considered that the level to which the ODP is able to do this is constrained by resources and time restraint.
3. Nonmaleficence – all treatments involve some harm, even if minimal, but the harm should not be disproportionate to the benefits of the treatment; for example, intubation may result in a sore throat (harm). However, this is outweighed by the need to secure a patent airway and ventilate the patient. Nonmaleficence requires the ODP to refrain from doing harm or prevent any action that could cause harm.

    The premise of these two principles should not be confused; beneficence is about being active in doing good. Nonmaleficence is about actively preventing harm. These principles are difficult to uphold in all situations because there are times when even the need to gain intravenous access can be problematic, causing harm although ultimately it does benefit the patient.
4. Justice – this principle is based around fairness and rights ensuring equality for all to healthcare. Equality for all in receiving treatment and access to services is notional, as it is more about treating people as individuals and recognizing their differences and needs. The principle for the ODP means that they plan and provide care irrespective of the socio-economic status, race, gender or religion and that they ensure that they make the best use of resources and allocation available to them within the confines afforded to them. The ODP may not have power or control over the access and distribution over resources, but they do have a duty of care and responsibility to inform the appropriate people of any shortfall and follow this up.

**Stop and think**

Ethical dilemmas are created when competing values arise within teams. The principle of autonomy can often conflict with the principle of nonmaleficence. Allowing someone a choice within the periop-erative environment can give rise to an issue of safety and therefore the patient is unable to be self-determining. This may require some intervention or restraint.

An example of this is where a patient who has an indwelling catheter on arrival at theatre wants it removed and is making an attempt to remove it themselves. The patient is being irrational, but the ODP is trying to explain that it is not in their best interest, as well as restraining them from removing it. However, a member of the care team feels that the patient is not being listened to and that their views should be respected. The member of the team may disagree from a personal viewpoint and this can give rise to conflict – presenting that they are upholding the patient's right to choose. It is essen-tial that conflicts are explored but it is also essential to reach a compromise when the espoused values cannot be achieved within a given situation. It is also important that the relationship should not suffer but give rise to respect from sharing those conflicts. Timely discussion is paramount.

Using an example of your own from experience discuss how you would respond to a team member who was expressing their feelings on the right for the patient to choose? Consider the implications and how you would handle the situation?

The four principle ethics approach has remained unchallenged within the field of healthcare for many years. There is an emerging approach called virtue ethics that rejects the principles for resolving moral problems but instead relies on terms such as honesty, courage, compassion, tolerance, integrity, fairness and self-control. Some feel that this has gained in importance because of the dissatisfaction with some aspects of mainstream theories of ethics (Oakley, 1998).

The theories have been presented to give the practitioner an overview and further reading is encouraged and recommended to gain further insight.

### An ethical rule approach

In 2007 Newham and Hawley introduced the concept of ethical rules around two aspects of ethics that are often referred to as principles. However, unlike a principle, the ethical rules of confidentiality and truthfulness do not have to be adhered to providing there are sufficient grounds to support this.

The ethical rule of confidentiality requires ODPs to refrain from disclosing information to others as well as ensuring records are kept safe and in confidence. It should be remembered that this rule does continue after the patient has died. There are exceptions to the rule where it is in the patient's best interest that information they have informed you about is shared. The need to share information in healthcare should always be on a 'need to know' basis and not purely for interest.

The ethical rule of veracity (truthfulness) is about truth telling and honesty preserving the trust in the relationship with the healthcare practitioner. The practitioner needs to inform the patient about the care they will receive and this must be truthful, while remembering that the ODP should only discuss such information that is within their scope of practice. The patient relies on the practitioner being honest so that they can make a rational decision and act autonomously. However, if a patient was to ask an ODP in the anaesthetic room, 'Can you tell if I will have a painful jaw after the opera-tion as a number of my friends have suffered with this and no one has mentioned it to me?', the ODP may choose to refrain from answering this question in a straightforward manner. Instead, the ODP may inform the patient that they are unaware of this even though there has been a high incident of this lately, so as not to cause undue anxiety for the patient. The ODP has a responsibility to pass on the patients' concerns to the anaesthetist prior to induction so that their concerns can be dealt with. The patient may need prompting by the ODP to ask the anaesthetist to discuss the matter that concerns them as too often they feel that they do not want to make a fuss. The matter will need to be handled sensitively and some information may be withheld at this point as it may be felt insensitive at that stage of the proceedings and may not be of benefit to the patient.

The theories and rules are brief and it may seem that no one theory is best, but that does not mean they do not have value. The theories can be used to resolve real ethical dilemmas and conflict by looking at differing viewpoints, which will hopefully support and structure future issues.

### Stop and think

Before moving on it would be useful to reflect on your own beliefs and ideas in relation to your practice. Ask yourself:

- What are the agreed standards of ethical practice in the perioperative environment?
- What role does the ODP play in ethical practice within the team?
- What are the two most frequent ethical dilemmas you experience in your working practice?

## Values

Values play a significant role in the codes of professional practice. Henry stated that 'the stronger the ethos is in ethical values within a culture of an institution, the more distinctive the institution will be' (Henry et al., 1992: 123). It is important to explore values and codes of professional practice as these are fundamental to the relationships within teams. The guiding standards for ODPs can be found within the codes of professional practice, but first it is important to understand what values actually are.

### What are values?

According to Fry and Johnstone there are differences between personal and professional values. Personal values are 'individual's beliefs, attitudes, standards and ideals that guide behaviour and how an individual experiences life'; and professional values 'are the ultimate standards that have been agreed to and are expected to be upheld by a professional group' (Fry and Johnstone, 2002: 6).

You may share your personal values with family, friends or other social groups, who may have values particular to you. These values emerge from your background, experiences and sense of self. Many values stay constant in your life while others will change and develop over time. Values are often about ideals and there is an element of compromise and change that takes place. These changes can take place through reflection, experience or pressure to align your values with others in a social context.

Professional values are ones held by that profession. The professional values for ODPs are set out by the Health and Care Professions Council (HCPC Standards of Performance, Conduct and Ethics (2012). These standards are written in such a way that they are able to be interpreted by all those professional groups regulated by the HCPC.

Although there are many professions working collaboratively within the perioperative environment that have their own codes and standards, they all have underpinning core values such as:

- respecting the individual patient;
- obtaining informed consent before any treatment or care;
- protecting any confidential information;
- co-operating with others on a team;
- maintaining professional knowledge and competence;
- being trustworthy;
- acting in a way where you minimize or identify any risk to the patient.

Complex issues can arise when the values held by a particular individual or group come into conflict with those of their employing organization.

The NHS provides a clear set of values that sets out how professionals working within the organization should behave, and the approach they should take. The Department of Health produced *The Handbook to the NHS Constitution* for England (2013) sets out six values that provide a common ground for co-operation to achieve shared aspirations to the public, patients and staff. The independent sector will have similar guidance for shared values and in the main they will not be too dissimilar to the NHS. The six areas do correlate with professional codes and guidance and they also encourage a more participative engagement of the patient. But the aspiration of the NHS values, respecting the rights of patients to be more participative, means that the patient needs not only to be informed, but also to have the confidence to engage more. The ODP should recognize that not all patients want to be fully engaged when coming to the operating theatre as often they 'would rather not know what is about to happen to them'. Their individual needs should be respected, while at the same time communication must be maintained so that they feel they can ask at any time about their care. The ODP needs to recognize that in the perioperative environment participation can be limited due to a context of the care being delivered.

### Stop and think

Practitioners can face dilemmas when the choices patients make are incongruent with the practitioners' own personal and professional values. For example, imagine a patient has decided to reject the treatment they have been offered that can potentially prolong their life. They do not want family members knowing about the treatment, even though one of the family members could be a donor. The practitioner needs to weigh up how respecting the person's request for confidentiality (autonomy) and the potential to treatment would benefit them (beneficence). It can be uncomfortable for the practitioner involved as it may be something they cannot understand and they will find their personal and professional values being challenged. The practitioner needs to respect the individuals' decision and their right to choose what information is shared and with whom; also that they can decide what intervention they want or do not want – self-determination.

Reflect on the scenario above and discuss the balancing of the values that have been expressed. Now using an example of your own experience, whether as a patient or colleague, explore some of the value judgements that are involved, remembering that context is important. Does any of this conflict with your personal values? How would you resolve the situation in an ethical professional way?

The theories and guiding standards of our professional values structure our professional behaviour but there are many other factors that conflict and create professional ethical dilemmas. The following section explores a number of situations in practice where the ODP may face dilemmas.

## Ethics in practice

It is helpful to explore and reflect upon real-life situations where ODPs may face difficult and complex dilemmas. This will help professional development regarding the ethical aspect of practice.

### Resuscitation

Resuscitation refers to reviving a person by the process of sustaining life of the vital systems such as the respiratory, cardiac and correcting the acid-base balance. Often this takes place in an emergency situation and little time is given for discussion on whether the person wanted to be resuscitated or not. All patients have a right to refuse treatment or resuscitation but unless there has been a clear briefing of this request, the ODP will be unaware of their wishes. It is important that if these are the patient's wishes they should be relayed to all those who are caring for them. There are situations that may override this mainly due to the timing and circumstances such as when a patient expresses '*in the event of their heart stopping they do not wish to be resuscitated*'. These are extremely difficult situations and in practice the practitioner and colleagues will always act in the patient's best interest.

### Do not attempt resuscitation (DNAR)

These documents are often drawn up and placed in the patient's notes with the patient's consent form. There are some very good guidelines on how to prepare such a document by the Resuscitation Council UK (2009), although each hospital will have protocols that an ODP will need to understand.

A DNAR document should always be drawn up in advance following discussion with the patient and/or other family members and/or significant others. This empowers the patient and gives them autonomy, with a right to choose how they would like to be treated when least able to do so for themselves. It becomes complicated if a patient states that they wish to be resuscitated even when it is explained that to do so could result in their outcome being worse should they survive. However, doctors do have the right to refuse treatment to what they feel is both futile and burdensome (Schwartz et al., 2002). The ODP needs to be aware of the Association of Anaesthetists for Great Britain and Northern Ireland (AAGBI) guidelines for managing a patient with a DNAR decision for the perioperative period. It states that 'all theatre staff should be made aware of the DNAR management option of the patient throughout their time in the theatre suite and recovery area.' (AAGBI, 2009: 22). It also stresses that the anaesthetist and surgeon should be available throughout to enable shared responsibility of any decisions to be made. The DNAR should be clearly communicated to the post-anaesthetic staff and the management option remains in place until transferred back to the ward. It is paramount that all analgesia and fluids are reviewed in the postoperative phase with the patient and carers.

Unfortunately, a number of cases have arisen where the DNAR has been placed in the notes by a medical practitioner but has not been discussed with patients or others and this has led to relatives questioning the care interventions and being upset.

## Refusal of blood

No two ethical issues are the same, due to the patient, the condition and how this can change so quickly, and this is especially true in the operating theatre. It is usually possible to adjust the planned care for a patient who is a Jehovah Witness to avoid the need for a blood transfusion. However, in an emergency situation, where there may be the need for transfusion due to complications, and the decision to refuse a life-saving blood transfusion may cause conflict in the practitioner who must do good (beneficence) and cause no harm (nonmaleficence) while respecting the autonomy of the patient and to give them the right to choose to refuse treatment. The values of the healthcare team and the patient may be incongruent but the patient has a right to refuse even life-saving treatment. When it comes to the parent making the choice for their child in such circumstances, clinicians can seek a court decision to gain a temporary ward of the court removing the rights of the parents to withhold consent to a blood transfusion. This is a long process and one that does impact on the relationship with the doctor and the health team. Consideration needs to be given to the implications of the effect of such a decision and the long-term impact on the child and their family. According to Veatch, treating a patient when there was a refusal of treatment violated peoples' rights to make a self-sacrifice of expression from what they believed in and of which they were members (Veatch, 2000).

### Ethical decision making

It is invaluable in practice that ODPs think through issues and problems especially where it involves an ethical element. If these situations were rehearsed either by posing a scenario or by reflecting on a 'real' situation it can contribute towards developing ethical thinking in practice, so to structure this thinking the use of a framework of questions can be of benefit. Using the theories and approaches discussed can support the discussion and offer support to resolving conflict within the professional environment.

An ethical dilemma occurs when we are forced to choose between two different actions, and choosing one action will mean that another good is sacrificed; for example, if you promised your friend that you would attend her oncology appointment with her, but on the day you receive a call from your mother who has had a serious accident and is on her way to the hospital. This dilemma may seem easy – you would go to your mother in the hospital. However, you may become torn between your obligations to your friend, and her life-threatening problem and your mother. Various factors may influence your thinking; for example, do you get along with your mother or do you break a promise to attend the hospital with your friend? The situation facing you is about making a choice between keeping a promise (a moral good) and attending to the care of your mother in hospital (a moral good). If this is a personal choice, we can usually just think about the issue, weighing up the goods and the potential harm each option may present, and can make this decision relatively easily. We do not have to stop and think as we go with a gut instinct. In professional practice our ethical decisions mean we are accountable to many others and the impact can be wide so we need to think through the issues to make these choices.

To support the ODP the proposal of a framework of questions has been developed to guide ethical decision making. The framework has been informed by some key organizations such as the Markkula Centre for Applied Ethics and the UK Clinical Ethics Network (UKCEN) but they have been placed in the context for the ODP in the perioperative environment although they can be transferred to any clinical area.

## A framework of questions for ODPs

Developing good ethical decision making requires compassion and awareness of ethical issues. By using this approach you can look at the ethical aspects of a decision, weighing up the significance of any actions and how they impact on practise. Having such an approach can support growth of the individual and the team. When practised regularly, the method becomes so familiar that it can be worked through without having to refer to all the questions separately.

The more complex the situation, the more you need to rely on discussion and dialogue with others about the dilemma, therefore reflection on the problem, supported by the insights and different perspectives of others, will provide valuable learning.

### A framework of questions to support and resolve ethical issues

- Have you identified the ethical issue? Do you have all the facts about the situation? Who are the individuals within the team that are involved and affected? In what way are they affected and are there any conflicts?
- What are the ethical issues? Be specific and see if they relate to the HCPC standards, other professionals codes that have been breached or are there organizational aspects of concern?
- What are the actual principles that are of concern? Is this related to professional behaviour; competence; due care; integrity; confidentiality or other?
- Are there any internal procedures you need to consider such as policies, procedures or the need to escalate to senior staff? Is there a whistle-blowing policy and/or raising and escalating concerns?
- Consideration needs to be given to organizational guidelines and processes, legal and regulatory aspects, and consequences of the issue. Has this been a long-term issue?
- Make notes and document your thought process and timeline as these help to clarify and justify your course of action.

The framework of questions appears formal but its purpose is to create a logical approach. By taking this approach it gives a sense of order and sequencing that can contribute towards developing ethical practice. Many practitioners who face ethical situations, or a situation in which others are involved, often do so as a novice in their early professional career. This is in part due to no two situations being exactly the same. To develop towards mastery it requires a deliberate approach by using the above framework of questions, debriefs and case scenario to support the ODP on their recall and reflection on the given ethical dimensions of the situation. Ethical theories help us communicate and in doing this the ODP can discuss issues with others, and hear their perspectives using a common language.

### Advocacy

It is important that in healthcare the patient can feel supported and able to express their wishes and this is where the role of advocacy plays a part. Advocacy is about supporting an individual or group to enable them to express their views or representing these on their behalf. In practice it presents a continuum that may vary depending on the healthcare environment. In the perioperative environment patients often feel vulnerable and the expectation is that the professional will act in their best interest.

The role of advocacy within the perioperative environment is different due to insufficient time of building a relationship prior to the care intervention. There are a number of characteristics that can be drawn from literature, but for an ODP there is still no clear description of the role of an advocate within the perioperative environment. There are four characteristics that fit well with the role and they include:

- informing the patient and to promote informed consent;
- empower the patient and protect autonomy;
- protect the rights and interests of patients where they cannot protect their own;
- ensure patients have fair access to available resources.

These are not contentious and are often seen as part of the overall aspect of being a professional within this and other related environments. However, multidisciplinary working involves complex interactions between different professionals and ensuring there is a common purpose. This is often achieved in good practice by briefing and debriefing sessions.

The crucial time when a patient requires an advocate is when they are confused and frightened, incompetent or unconscious. It is therefore paramount that the ODP realizes that it is not about speaking and representing their views, which are often unknown, but should be about protecting the rights and interest of patients who cannot protect their own. It is about ensuring the patient has a clear understanding and is enabled to consult with others expressing their wishes as appropriate thereby protecting their autonomy while ensuring they receive adequate resources to meet their needs.

These factors can cause tension when patients' desires are not conducive to a safe delivery of care, such as wanting to get off the bed or trolley. Sufficient resources can also cause undue tension. The practitioner needs to ensure that these shortfalls or requirements are communicated effectively within the organization, especially to those who have responsibility for the wider remit for quality and governance of the care delivered.

It needs to be made clear that representing the patient's wishes is the best way to protect and maintain their integrity and therefore autonomy. This is not performing an advocacy role but acting as a professional who is committed to the duty of care and adhering to their professional standards. If the professional portrays what they perceive as the patient's wishes, however well intended, they need to be aware that they may be acting in a paternalistic manner that could be interpreted as being coercive.

Some ODPs working in advanced practice may have a more long-term relationship with a patient and this will change the idea and approach of an advocate role as the relationship develops. Compliance of the regulatory body's requirements and that of the patient's wishes is paramount. However, like other healthcare professionals, there may be times when your own professional judgement and that of the patients will not be in harmony. The advocate's role must protect and be representative of the patient's needs and values. It is the responsibility of all practitioners to work within the parameters and scope of their practice including any further education and training required to develop their understanding and to benefit the patient.

## Conclusion

This chapter has only given the reader an insight to this vast subject, and wider reading is highly recommended. It is paramount that ODPs understand the impact the ethical dimension has on their practice and, when working alongside other professionals, they must not be the passive participant in ensuring the delivery of ethical practice. The ODP has become an essential member of the team with an increase in role and responsibility both in and outside of the perioperative environment, and this has given rise to needing clarity and a broader understanding of ethics in their practice. The HCPC provide a standard framework by which the ODP is required to behave, but a greater understanding of ethical theories and values in conjunction with these codes will help with the ODP's development as an ethical practitioner.

The integration of the 'four principle' ethics approach within the utilitarian ethos of the NHS is often based around the consequences of actions; that is, weighing up which action would be least harmful and of most benefit to a particular individual, and which action would benefit most people or the use of resources most efficiently. The fundamental concept is that the right action is that which produces the greatest balance of good over evil (principle of utility).

It is fair to say that all professionals involved in care delivery within the perioperative environment must collaborate with each other for the patient and the wider health community in a manner that respects the ethical principles of professionalism and healthcare. Healthcare organizations have the obligation to establish processes that identify new procedures or practices that can be seen to be of benefit to the patient. However, only with the co-operation of all the healthcare teams can the system produce optimal outcomes and value for the individual patient.

## Key points

- How ethical theories guide current practice.
- Structure on how to deal with ethical dilemmas.
- What it means to be an ethical practitioner.
- An understanding of personal and professional values.
- Ethics as part of the practitioners practice.

## References and further reading

Association of Anaesthetists for Great Britain and Northern Ireland (AAGBI) (2009) *Do Not Attempt Resuscitation (DNAR): Decisions in the Perioperative Period*. London: AAGBI.

Beauchamp, T.L. and Childress, J.F. (2001) *Principles of Biomedical Ethics* (5th edn). Oxford: Oxford University Press.

Department of Health (DH) (2013) *The Handbook to the NHS Constitution for England*. London: DH. Available online at www.gov.uk/...data/.../the-nhs-constitution-for-england (accessed 20 August 2013).

Fry, S. and Johnstone, M. (2002) *Ethics in Nursing Practice* (2nd edn). Malden, MA: Blackwell Science.

Henry, C., Drew, J., Anwar, N., Campbell, G. and Benoit- Asselman, D. (1992) 'The EVA Project: University of Central Lancashire', in Henry, C. (ed.) (1995) *Professional Ethics and Organisational Change in Education and Healthcare* (p. 13). London: Edward Arnold.

Kant, I. (1964) *Groundwork of the Metaphysical of Morals*. New York: Harper & Row.

Markkula Centre for Applied Ethics. Available online at http://www.scu.edu/ethics (accessed 25 August 2013).

Mills, J.S. (1867) *Utilitarianism*. London: Longmans (reprint 1967).

Newham, R.A. and Hawley, G. (2007) 'The relationship to ethics to philosophy', in Hawley, G. (ed.) *Ethics In Clinical Practice: An Interprofessional Approach*. Harlow: Pearson Education.

Oakley, J. (1998) 'A virtue approach to ethics', in Kushe, H. and Singer, P. (eds) *A Companion of Ethics*. Oxford: Blackwell.

Resuscitation Council UK (2009) *Recommended Standards for Recording 'Do not attempt resuscitation' (DNAR) Decisions*. Available online at www.resus.org.uk (accessed 15 August 2013).

Schwatz, L., Preece, P.E. and Hendry, R.A. (2002) *Medical Ethics: A Case Based Approach*. Edinburgh: Saunders.

UK Clinical Ethics. Available online at http://www.ukcen.net (accessed 25 August 2013).

Veatch, R. (2000) 'Dr does not know best. why in the new century physicians must stop trying to benefit the patient', *Journal of Medicine and Philosophy*, 25 (6): 701–72.

# 8 Reflection for Operating Department Practitioners

## Penny Joyce

**Key topics**

- Reflection in operating department practice
- Reflective practice as an everyday occurrence
- Reflective professional practice

- Types of reflection – reflection on and in action
- Ways to reflect
- Consequences of reflection
- Toolkit for reflection

## Introduction

Reflection is an important human activity in which people recapture their experience, think about it, mull over and evaluate it. It is this working with experience that is important in learning (Boud et al., 1985: 43). Reflection is an integral part of our lives, whether a student Operating Department Practitioner (ODP) or an experienced practitioner or simply as part of everyday activities. It is more than a buzzword; it presents an opportunity to draw your thoughts together, gives focus and demonstrates learning. Frequently used in education through a structured approach, it allows students to move from a simple descriptive framework to more complex processes that allow deeper, more critical thinking; more informally, it is part of everyday activities, human development and interactions. This chapter explores the relevance to learners; this includes pre-registration students but also acknowledges that at any stage of our career we are all learners to some degree, and therefore must consider the opportunities and tools for learning through reflection, reflective writing, professional development and the more analytical and critical aspects of reflection.

Without doubt reflection is seen as an essential component of improving professional practice for health professionals. Schön (1983) is a name synonymous with reflection in healthcare, but he was not the first to provide evidence for this. In fact Schön did not particularly write about healthcare professionals, but he along with Boud et al. (1985) and Dewey (1933) have been among the most influential in developing reflection within healthcare education, particularly in nursing (Jasper, 2003). Schön remains at the core of contemporary thinking in relation to professionals' application of reflective action and thinking. The significance of his work still influences many training and education programmes with the philosophy of theory and practice being tightly integrated as a core component.

Dewey (1933) defined reflection as an active persistent and careful consideration of any belief or supposed form of knowledge in the light of the grounds that support it and the further conclusion it reaches. Boud et al. (1985) take a different perspective and define it as a more generic term for those intellectual and effective activities in which individuals engage to explore their experiences in order to lead to a new understanding and appreciation. They view reflection from the learner's point of view. They discuss the relationship of the reflective process and the learning experience against what the learner can do.

## Relevance to ODPs

The Health and Care Professions Council (HCPC) *Standards of Proficiency for Operating Department Practitioners* state in standard 11 '. . . be able to reflect on and review practice' (2014). In addition, the College of Operating Department Practitioners (CODP) clearly articulate within the professional curriculum the need for reflection and the ability to reflect as key outcomes for ODPs (CODP, 2011: 15, 21, 23) in order to develop and promote safe and effective patient care. In a small-scale ODP cohort study it was shown that student learning is reliant on an experiential approach, in this case simulation, and that reflection is a vehicle for this in order to effect cognitive change (Joyce, 2011). ODPs need to develop strong interpersonal skills in order to facilitate patient care in the operating theatre environment; this along with self-awareness and the ability to directly influence or change practice to ensure positive outcomes in all aspects of perioperative care are key skills. Reflective practice facilitates the development of these key skills by encouraging ODPs to understand the events or experiences that happen and through analysis come to a deeper understanding or clarity about them, and therefore inform future and evolving practice.

## Reflective practice as an everyday occurrence

The professional and regulatory position clearly presents the relevance of this topic for ODPs, but both as practitioners and learners, reflection is simply embedded within everyday life. 'Experiences' happen all the time, consciously and subconsciously; we think about what happened and 'relive' that experience even if done later or not taken any further than this descriptive process. We rarely take the time to analyse the routine and everyday experiences we have and ask ourselves:

- What have I just done/experienced?
- Why did I do it that way?
- Have I done it before, did the last time influence me this time?
- Could I have done it any differently?
- How will I do it next time?

**Stop and think**

Think about some of the everyday experiences you have encountered in the last few weeks; for example, washing, shopping, socializing, reading, driving, eating and getting to work/studies. Now ask yourself the prompt questions above – have you considered this process of reflective learning?

Take the example of 'washing' as portrayed by a student who is currently living away from home at university. This is their first experience of selecting washing products such as washing powder, liquid or fabric softener. When reflecting on the brand of washing powder they chose, they stated that the choice they made was the same brand they had witnessed being used at home and it was considered 'very good'. They therefore made the choice based on the influence from a previous experience. The student could have bought any brand, maybe gone for the cheapest, biggest pack or best value for money.

These are all aspects that may influence the student in the future. This analogy could be applied to many everyday aspects of life – the bread we buy, the beer we drink or the drive to work; we do not have the time to sit back and reflect in a structured way for every routine experience we have. Jasper

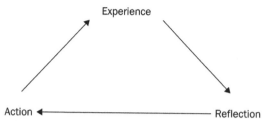

**Figure 8.1** The reflective experience, reflection and action (ERA) cycle.
*Source:* Jasper (1999: 2, fig. 1.1); used with permission from Cengage Learning EMEA Ltd

(1999) explains this process as having three components that make up the cycle of experience, reflection and action (see ERA cycle, Figure 8.1) and presents a very simple framework for reflection that suggests that we learn from thinking about things that have happened to us. This applies equally to everyday life a well as through developing professional practice.

This process of managing the 'routine' has made us effective in daily activities, but as you gain experience and watch others, by observing things done differently, so you will begin to change the way you do things. Even if after experimenting in this way you revert to the way you have always done it, that decision will be based on reflective thinking and reflective practice, albeit from a passive stance.

Learners really demonstrate their learning through reflection, and it is a tool they are introduced to early in their education. Johns (1995) notes that reflection enables the practitioner to assess understand and learn through their experiences. The development of professional expertise is more than a collection of knowledge and skills; it is the integration of knowledge and skills appropriate to each unique situation that is faced (Eraut, 1994). It is a personal process that usually results in some change in their perspective of a situation or creates new learning. The connection between reflection and learning has been developed by a number of educational theorists, one who is key and most well known is Kolb (1984) and his work on the cycle of experiential learning (Figure 8.2) that has been the foundation of many other models for reflective practice. Kolb's theory directs us to recall and observe the experience we want to learn from, reflect on that experience and in doing so describe

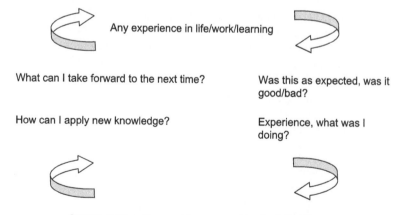

**Figure 8.2** Learning from experiences.
*Source:* adapted from Kolb (1984)

that experience. Once described you can then try and make sense (analyse), what happened, why it happened and perhaps explore other theories relating to the experience (read around the subject, look at the evidence base for example), and draw on your own theories or ideas about it. This process will allow you to gain a greater understanding and as Kolb proposes you will frame some action from the process – this action being the learning.

Kolb (1984) proposes four phases of experiential learning, which are essentially reflective:

1.  The experience.
2.  The reflection on what has happened then takes place: 'Was it a good, poor or mediocre performance?' 'What did I learn from the experience – I know what I am doing or need to learn more?'
3.  This phase is 'abstract conceptualization', a time when the student will attempt to understand why they went wrong/did well or could have improved. They also start to consider 'next time I'll . . .'
4.  The final stage is application of the knowledge/skills learned from the experience.

Of course this is a cyclical process so it never really comes to an end; it simply continues to evolve as the lifelong learner does, with each new experience, knowledge and theory increasing learning at each revolution. Therefore reflection is associated with a deeper approach to learning that allows integration with existing knowledge and skills. Sandars identified reflection as often not being integrated into the curriculum, seen as a 'bolt on extra' (2009: 693). In this situation both tutors and students are in danger of seeing this as disconnected from the learning process that can result in poor engagement and is considered as a consequence of reflection later in the chapter.

For professional practice this cycle of learning is essential to develop our role as ODPs, the learning from experience is constantly being fed back into our practice and building knowledge and experience every time. This learning process is therefore not just looking back, but as a spiral of learning from which experience develops, facilitating planning for further development and new experiences.

## Reflective professional practice

Reflection places value on an experience and offers the opportunity to show where learning and changes have taken place. This will encourage you to pose and answer key questions about your experiences such as why it happened, when it happened and how it happened. Therefore, this gives you an opportunity to place your experiences into the context of your professional practice and to record the learning that comes out of such experiences whether a student or qualified ODP at any stage in their career development. An important aspect of becoming, or being a practitioner, is to develop the ability to reflect on everyday experiences in a meaningful way, and in a variety of settings. The reasons why you may choose to reflect can include:

*   continuing professional development;
*   learning from specific incidents;
*   sharing good practice;
*   developing new ideas;
*   identifying personal learning needs;
*   to learn a new task/skill/technique;
*   explore personal feelings;
*   make sense of an incident/experience;
*   demonstrate ability to others;
*   problem solve;
*   support decision making;
*   debrief self and others;
*   anticipate (reflect before action).

These are just some areas, and the list is not exhaustive but clearly reflective practice is a framework for practitioners and aspiring practitioners to learn from their experiences. In the perioperative environment anticipation (reflection before action) is a key skill; for example, when assisting with a potentially difficult airway the ODP may reflect upon similar previous experiences to inform their actions.

The notion of 'experience' is worth considering here. A tendency to consider an experience as 'critical' in terms of complexity, urgency or consequence has often been portrayed, but it can simply relate to any life event however routine and simple that contributes to development. The outcomes of such events may have been positive, negative or completely neutral. It may also be a series of events or an accumulation of experience over time on which you choose to reflect. So the term 'experience' should be held to the broadest of meanings – it could well be a one-off event, or a process over time of experiences, skills and knowledge. The trigger for such reflections can be derived from experiences that:

- have gone really well;
- went badly wrong;
- you did not understand;
- you feel really good about;
- made you feel uncomfortable/sad/angry;
- you have had feedback on your role/performance;
- you want to share with others.

It can be seen here that reflective practice carries multiple meanings both in terms of why to reflect and what to reflect on. This will always be individual to the practitioner, and as a learner or practitioner the more formal and structured approached is usually determined by explicit criteria in their curricula. Smyth (1992: 285) suggests that 'reflection can mean all things to all people . . . it is used as a kind of umbrella or canopy term to signify something is good or desirable'.

There is a danger for learners and practitioners that reflection can become a ritual, sometimes artificial in the desire to ensure that professional and regulatory bodies criteria to be a 'reflective practitioner' are met. Practices such as a checklist for reflection on practice placements, for example, can be mechanistic and lead learners and practitioners to be unaware of the consequences of reflection at times.

## Consequences of reflection

Reflective practice is widely acknowledged to be an essential foundation for professional development, and a tool for lifelong learning, and done well it is a valuable tool to explore, transform and progress practice. But it also raises some consequences, which need to be considered whether you are a registered ODP, a student, or delivering ODP education.

Teaching reflective practice raises two main concerns: first, the extent to which students are ready in their development to reflect appropriately; and second, the mandatory element of reflective practice by virtue of a pre-registration curriculum for example. Readiness to reflect can be problematic as learners by nature are novices in their professional field, so movement from the descriptive stage to the action (learning) stage needs to be carefully nurtured. Learners often are not aware of the issues to consider at the evaluation stage. If they are presented only with a checklist on which to reflect their learning from practice experience, it will become process driven and they will not develop the skills in which to consider what, why and how to reflect for any given experience. Finlay (2008: 16) suggests four guiding principles for educators:

- present reflective practice with care;
- provide adequate support, time, resources, opportunities and methods for reflection;

- develop (learners') skills of critical analysis;
- take proper account of the context of reflection.

The mandatory requirement of reflection in an ODP pre-registration programme can have the potential to make the process very false. Learners from other professions where reflection is assessed significantly have been found to adopt an approach to perform in order to pass (Hargreaves, 2004); Hobbs (2007: 413) more radically suggests 'reflection and assessment are incompatible'. However even with academically driven activities such as 'having to do reflection', they are widely acknowledged as valuable for deeper understanding.

Professional and ethical consequences are other aspects to be considered. Some of the ethical issues consist of confidentiality, informed consent, professional relationships, disclosure, misconduct, status of the records (if written/recorded reflection) and emotional impact.

So just as important as learning the ways and models to reflect, so is the wider context of sharing the risks and ensuring students are fully aware of the potential for conflicts of interest. Reflection can have a profound emotional effect to the reflector, it is essential to be aware of this risk to cause harm, and educators including clinical mentors need to be sensitive to this issue. They may well find themselves outside of their level of expertise and need to ensure that when necessary the need to refer to an appropriate practitioner or expert may be necessary, as you might for any experience outside or beyond your scope of expertise (HCPC, 2012).

## Types of reflection – reflection on and in action

Schön (1983), who remains as one of the most influential writers, describes reflection in two main ways: reflection *on* action and reflection *in* action. Reflection *on* action is looking back after the event while reflection *in* action is happening during the event. In professional practice examples of reflecting *on* practice are thinking about an experience after it happened; judging how successful it was, what could you do better and so on. Fitzgerald (1994: 67) defines this as 'the retrospective contemplation of practice undertaken in order to uncover the knowledge used in practical situations, by analysing and interpreting the information recalled'.

This is usually the most common type of reflection for student ODPs to engage in as part of their studies and knowledge development; and for those new to reflection this is usually the starting point.

Reflection *in* action allows the ODP to redesign what they are doing while they are doing it. So, for example, while considering the suitability of DVT prophylaxis equipment for a particular patient they will be reassessing, the choice and how effective it is or might be while undertaking the task. This type of reflection is commonly associated with experienced practitioners and Greenwood (1993) suggests this is usually triggered by an unexpected result or even surprise in the experience/activity being undertaken. Schön's real contribution was to reveal how professionals cope with complex problems and the type of reflection that supports this, either reflection on or in action, identifying limitations and guiding future development.

The practitioner allows himself to experience surprise, puzzlement, or confusion in a situation which he finds uncertain or unique. He reflects on the phenomenon before him, and on the prior understandings which have been implicit in his behaviour. He carries out an experiment which serves to generate both a new understanding of the phenomenon and a change in the situation

(Schön 1983: 68)

However, an ODP's experiences in perioperative care are usually time critical; decisions need to be made and the time for reflection and consideration unrealistic. But what is evident is that despite not closely following a 'textbook' theme, as practitioners we do think things through and as every case is unique we do have to draw on the experiences that have gone before.

Reflecting on professional practice or undertaking reflection as an academic requirement in this way can help you to understand yourself as it may make your personal feelings; such as biases, expectations and beliefs far more evident to you. By understanding yourself in terms of learning, knowledge and personal feelings, it can support your studies and developing professional practice, as it will make you aware of potential assumptions that can be made almost automatically when you do not set out to reflect consciously on actions, or why you have done things a certain way.

## Ways to reflect

Essentially there are three ways to do this, as an individual, with another (such as mentor, peer or colleague) or as a group. The experience and what you hope to gain (learn) from the process will usually determine the way you choose to reflect and this may differ from occasion to occasion, and may consist of one or more ways for each experience.

Reflecting as an individual:

- Thinking through an experience (reflection on practice).
- Thinking back on an experience (reflection in practice).
- Reflective writing; for example, reflective reports/accounts/essays, learning logs, activity logs, diaries/journals, critical analysis, email, social networks.
- Reflecting with another; for example, talking through an experience with a peer/colleague, tutorial, clinical supervision, appraisal, presentation, email, social networks.
- Group reflection; for example, reflective group work/seminars/presentations, during/following role play/simulation, team debrief session, critical incident analysis

Reflecting on your own can be as simple as mulling over the experiences of the day on your way home or making entries to a diary or log of activities. Often this process will not develop beyond the descriptive so opportunities to really 'unpick' the events or turn the thoughts into action/learning are not realized. Reflective writing is a strategy that can be used for many purposes and does allow for a more thoughtful and structured approach to emerge. While it is far more prevalent in those who are undertaking some formal learning at any stage of their development (from a pre-registration student to advanced practitioner), it is undoubtedly a valuable way in which to become a 'consciously reflective practitioner' (Jasper, 2003: 143). It also forms a record of your activity and learning that could be used for evidence; for example, an assessment for a student, which will be considered later; or as a practitioner for your CPD evidence in an HCPC audit. As an example consider the case of an ODP who has undertaken a mentorship course. Mentorship, whether initial preparation for the role or updating, is commonly an activity for professional development as an ODP. To put this in context specifically for the HCPC audit process, an example of mentorship development is demonstrated against the HCPC standards for CPD.

Every two years a number of ODPs are selected for CPD audit; if selected you will need to submit a profile, HCPC will provide the template for this. The profile has five sections to it. Section 1 is simply your profession and unique CPD number. Section 2 is a brief summary of your current and aspirant role as appropriate therefore sections 1 and 2 set the context. Section 3 is a personal statement, which evaluates your CPD in relation to standards 3 and 4 by using the three stages of the ERA framework; *experience* being the mentorship course and by *reflecting* on this you will analyse how and why this has improved your practice and contributed to other service users. In your analysis you will *action* developments or opportunities for future practice and service delivery. The penultimate section 4 is the evidence submitted in support of the selected CPD being discussed, and finally section 5 is the list of all your CPD for the audit period; both of these are therefore the evidence for your standards. The key to presenting your CPD to HCPC if selected for audit is therefore via a reflective process on the value it has been to you. Figure 8.3 sets this in context by showing how the actual standards are met via a reflective process.

Less formally as part of your role as an ODP you will constantly be reflecting with others, but whether one-to-one or as a group it does bring some challenges as well as advantages. The advantages include: seeing things from another's perspective; using others as a sounding board for ideas; drawing on the expertise and experience of others; being asked questions you may not ask yourself; finding alternative actions and bringing a new context or objectivity to the fore. It is vital to also be aware of the challenges in reflecting with others and the need to have clear ground rules at the onset,

---

The first two standards relate to the 'experience' or 'what' (Borton, 1970).

**Standard 1: maintain a continuous, up to date and accurate record of their CPD activities.** This will be a list of all your CPD activities (section 5 of profile) during the audit period; *your mentorship course must be in this list.*

**Standard 2: demonstrate that their CPD activities are a mixture of learning activities relevant to current or future practice.** Your mentorship CPD could be a number of activities; for example, formal learning if you attended a course, online workshop to update, student feedback on your performance as a mentor, reading, peer evaluation or appraisal. *So if you look back your mentorship was probably a combination of these activities.*

The next 2 standards relate to 'reflection' or 'so what' – and also 'action' or 'now what' (Borton, 1970).

**Standard 3: seek to ensure that their CPD has contributed to the quality of their practice and service delivery.** You need to discuss here how your mentorship CPD has made you (or sought to make you) a better mentor. It may be that you are not yet a mentor but are planning to be, so a mentorship course, for example, may be part of the plan to achieve this goal. It might be essential updating in terms of the students' programme requirements, or you felt better time management or giving feedback were areas you needed to develop.

**Standard 4: seek to ensure that their CPD benefits the service user.** You need to identify your service users in the context of mentorship CPD; it is likely to be the students, but also the department, education manager or higher education institute (HEI) could be considered.

Standards 3 and 4 are the most critical and in-depth part of the profile and form section 3 of the HCPC template. This part demonstrates how the CPD has been of benefit to you and others. It is the value of the activities that counts, not so much what you have done, but what the experience and what you have learnt has done to develop you, so the reflective process is fundamental to this being achieved.

Standard 5 encapsulates the whole framework, presenting 'what, so what and now what' in context of the practitioner's role and development needs.

**Standard 5: upon request, present a written profile, which must be their own work and supported by evidence, explaining how they have met the standards for CPD.** From your list of CPD activities, select 3 or 4 samples to discuss in your profile, one of which could be your mentorship CPD. Authenticity of this will be assessed and evidence of the activities need to be provided. So, for example, you could include a mentorship certificate of achievement, student feedback (anonymous), literature critique, appraisal excerpt, peer evaluation or personal reflection.

**Figure 8.3** Example of integrating ERA into CPD standards.

which should include strict adherence to standards of professional conduct (HCPC, 2012) and awareness of the consequences such as confidentiality, disclosure and emotional control.

Increasingly reflecting with others is via engagement in a range of social networking channels such as Twitter, Facebook and Myspace, and any other number of communication media available now offers another avenue for reflective practice. Reflective and dialogic learning are clearly identified within eLearning pedagogy, the 'connectivist' learner being most likely to use a social network environment (Conole et al., 2010). Social networking is dominated by Facebook, with over 1.2 billion users; 98 per cent of 18–24 year olds using social media and 700 million minutes spent on Facebook alone every month (Social Education, 2012). It is therefore appropriate to consider its use in relation to reflective strategies in this chapter. Clearly, social networking media has revolutionized the way people connect socially. However, there are potential challenges, and therefore brings this warning that with such online activities the professional integrity of registered practitioners, and those aspiring to be registered could be called into question, as the blurring of personal and professional boundaries can easily occur. Even with the strictest privacy settings employed, any information placed on a social networking site is considered to have been put into the public domain and could be viewed by people other than the originator may have intended, therefore having the potential to breach confidentiality. Social networking used appropriately can be an asset to your communication networks, but you can innocently get caught up in a chain reaction to negative events that cross boundaries of professional and personal life all too easily.

## Toolkit for reflection

A number of frameworks (models) exist that will help ODP students and registrants structure reflection. Developing the skill of reflection will allow you to analyse and evaluate your learning experiences in greater depth and enable you to progress your practice or develop to more advanced study and learning. Three models are described in this section; two of which are among the most commonly and widely known models in healthcare (Jasper, 2003; Wigens, 2006) and the third offering an alternative view and one that may be more useful for reflecting in groups or with another. First, Gibbs' six-stage reflective cycle is described (Figure 8.4), followed by Borton's (1970) three-stage model (Figure 8.5) and finally the model suggested by Dyke (1990; Fig. 8.6) that proposes a different approach and is useful particularly in relation to reflection in groups.

Stage 1: Description – what happened?

Describe in detail the event you are reflecting on. Include things like where were you; who else was there; why were you there; what were you doing; what were other people doing; what was the context of the event; what happened; what was your part in this; what parts did the other people play; and what was the result?

Stage 2: Feelings – what were you thinking and feeling?

At this stage, try to recall and explore those things that were going on inside your head. Include:

- How you were feeling when the event started?
- What you were thinking about at the time?
- How did it make you feel?
- How did other people make you feel?
- How did you feel about the outcome of the event?
- What do you think about it now?

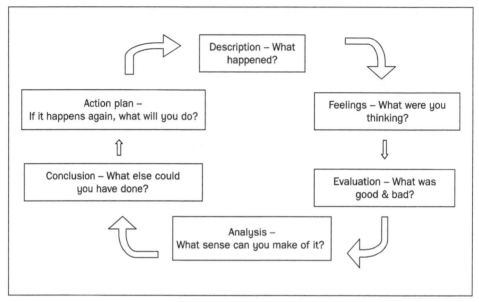

**Figure 8.4** Reflective cycle.
*Source:* adapted from Gibbs (1988)

Stage 3: Evaluation – what was good and bad about the experience?

Try to evaluate or make a judgement about what has happened. Consider what was good about the experience and what was bad about the experience or what did or did not go so well.

Stage 4: Analysis – what sense can you make of the experience?

Break down the event into its component parts so they can be explored separately. You may need to ask more detailed questions about the answers to the last stage. Include:

- What went well? Why do you think was?
- What did you do well?
- What did others do well?
- What went wrong or did not turn out how it should have done?
- In what way did you or others contribute to this?

Stage 5: Conclusion – what else could you have done?

This differs from the evaluation stage because you have explored the issue from a number of angles gaining further information on which to base your judgement. Remember the purpose of reflection is to learn from an experience. Without detailed analysis and honest exploration that occurs during all the previous stages, it is unlikely that all aspects of the event will be taken into account and therefore valuable opportunities for learning can be missed. During this stage you should ask yourself what you could have done differently.

Stage 6: Action Plan – if it happens again what would I do?

During this stage you should think about planning what you would do for next time – would you act differently or would you be likely to do the same? Do you need to get some training, gain new knowledge or learn about new equipment for example?

Here the cycle is notionally complete, but should the event occur again it will be the focus of another reflective cycle, and so to continually develop your professional practice. Gibbs is closely aligned to Kolb's learning cycle, and works on the premise of theory and practice continually enrich each other in a never-ending cycle. It is widely adopted in healthcare as a way to facilitate reflection and it is a model most ODPs are probably familiar with. However while it does offer a basic and clear way to structure reflection, it is also criticized in order to develop a broader and more critical reflexive approach (Jay and Johnson, 2002).

The second model is that of Borton (1970). It is a very simple model and certainly one that the author would advocate for the novice reflector. Borton provides a good starting point for student and registrant ODPs to make sense of firstly, and then make a response to real situations. Three key questions of *what, so what* and *now what?* They can be further supported with a number of cue questions for each:

*What?*

What happened?
What did I do?
What did others do?
What was I trying to achieve?
What was good or bad about the experience?

*So what?*

So why did it happen?
So what is the importance of this?
So what more do I need to know about this?
So what have I learned about this?

*Now what?*

Now what could I do next time?
Now what else do I need to do?
Now what might I do?
Now what might be the consequences of this action?

Figure 8.5 provides a fictitious example of an ODP student using Borton's model following a first placement where they had to reflect on one experience to demonstrate how HCPC professional standards could be illustrated.

As you can see this is a simple but effective way of formalizing a learning experience through reflection. Borton also tends to focus on reflection *on* action, looking back at an experience rather than using *in* action. A more experienced reflector my not opt for this model as a consequence. Emotions and feelings can be problematic and cause a novice reflector to get 'bogged down' in the initial stages, so this may be easier to start with than Gibbs, equally the deeper understanding of those emotions is an important part of the reflective process in order for learning to take place, the important part is to know yourself and understand how you learn best.

**Reflection on Foundation Placement**

**Introduction**

I am a first-year student Operating Department Practitioner (ODP) reflecting on the experience of my first placement, the Foundation Placement. Reflection is identified as a key way in which we can learn from experiences undertaken (Jasper, 2003). I will be using Borton's framework of reflection (Jasper, 2003); this provides a simple logical structure to focus on my learning and development and allows for a greater understanding of the experiences (Ghaye, 2005).

I will use the three prompt questions from Borton's model – what, so what and now what (Jasper, 2003). My reflection will incorporate the use of evidence to support practice and make reference to professional standards where appropriate.

**What?**

The placement is a four-week introductory phase of my clinical experience, during which time I had eight outcomes to achieve that focused on communication and health and safety areas. These were all achieved and I have selected just one specific experience to reflect on. In my third week I went with my mentor to do a preoperative visit to a patient due in theatre later that day. The patient was sat by her bed chatting to her husband. My mentor introduced herself and allowed me to do the same, at which point she tactfully interjected and took over the conversation.

**So what?**

When I introduced myself to the patient I explained I was a student and would also be present during her surgery; at the time I had started to say the actual operation, which is when my mentor carefully took over the conversation. After the visit my mentor explained that unless consent has been given to discuss any aspect of personal information or surgery in front of family or relatives, it is a breach of confidentiality (Health and Care Professions Council (HCPC), 2014). The HCPC *Standards of Conduct, Performance and Ethics* (2012) also highlight the need for every patient to be dealt with individually and respectfully; always acting in the patient's best interests. The intervention from my mentor ensured the patient was not compromised in any way, but also protected me from breaching confidentiality that I had not realized was so easy to do.

**Now what?**

Evaluating this event has increased my awareness of patient confidentiality, consent, data protection and identifying situations where this can so easily be breached, and not to make assumptions about what a close relative may know or not know. If a similar situation arises again I will be able to make an informed decision about gaining consent or considering options to ensure I maintain confidentiality (HCPC, 2012).

**Conclusion**

I have reflected on one event from my foundation placement; the structured process of a framework such as Borton's (Jasper, 2003) has allowed me to analyse the situation constructively and consider the professional issues in relation to this. I have recognized the development needs arising from this, which is an essential skill to progress as an accountable practitioner.

**References**

Ghaye, T. (2005) *Developing the Reflective Healthcare Team*. Oxford: Blackwell Publishing.

Health and Care Professions Council (HCPC) (2014) *Standards of Proficiency – Operating Department Practitioners*. London: HCPC.

Health and Care Professions Council. (2012) *Standards of Conduct, Performance and Ethics*. London: HCPC.

Jasper, M. (2003) *Beginning Reflective Practice: Foundations in Nursing and Healthcare*. Cheltenham: Nelson Thornes.

Wood, J. (2004) 'Clinical supervision'. *British Journal of Perioperative Nursing*, 14 (4): 151–56.

**Figure 8.5** Example of student using Borton in structured reflection.

## Critical reflection

While the Kolb, Gibbs and Borton models are familiar to ODP students and qualified practitioners alike, and are evaluated as useful learning tools, there is a concern of limiting development in critical reflection. Hull et al. (2005) challenge Kolb and Gibbs as representing a false picture, suggesting they do not reflect the real world that does not necessarily act so systematically and analyse each state on each occasion. Joyce (2011) found student ODPs frequently reflected together; more widely perioperative practitioners are engaging in team briefs and debriefs on a regular basis as part of the safer surgical initiative (World Health Organization (WHO), 2009), and it seems a weakness in encouraging the use of models such as those above is that it promotes individual reflection because it fails to engage ODPs more socially for collective reflection. This was the argument of Guille and Young (1998) who suggest that the social context is a key part of reflection in reflexive learning. Reflexivity/reflexive are frequently used words in connection with professional and personal development. Reynolds (1998) suggests four characteristics that clearly distinguish critical reflection from reflection:

- question assumptions;
- social not individual focus;
- analysis of relations;
- emancipation.

So, when an ODP critically reflects, they do far more than just looking back *on* or reflecting *in* an experience and unpicking the events; but they also look at the wider environment in which they are situated. This will allow them to consider the social stance and even power or influences exercised by the organization through its networks and wider relationships. While often they cannot impose transformational change or action at organizational level, it does encourage the practitioner to not be inhibited by such barriers to change as, for example, '. . . this is the way things are done here' culture.

Dyke (2009) offers an alternative framework for experiential learning, which is far more flexible than those already, discussed. As with other frameworks or models the ODP is still encouraged to include the theory, what they know; how this is applied, the experience itself; and reflect on these to inform future practice, but Dyke's model (2009: 306) does not rely on sequential steps or conforming to any direction, there are no arrows and therefore no order of events, which would support the developing student to learn more effectively, and importantly, recognizes the need to reflect with others.

Learning is often reliant on an experiential approach and reflection is a vehicle for this. But we need to consider whether the strategy used is restrictive in much the same way in clinical practice when applying a number of clinical algorithms to be ritually followed, offering a model of reflection is probably adhered to in the same way. Figure 8.6 is adapted from Dyke's original model, which demonstrated a lack of order and conformity without straight and regimented lines to follow in the more traditional frameworks seen earlier. If the signposts that suggest direction and sequence were removed as Dyke suggests, then the process will become more fluid, more critical and potentially of greater benefit to both the practitioner and students as they reflect with others in a team. My adaptation of this (Figure 8.6) shows the four aspects randomly connected but maybe of differing importance (size) with the central tenet being the opportunity to *reflect with others*. This is imperative for ODPs as teamwork is such an important player for perioperative practice.

### Stop and think

Consider an experience in the past week in your professional practice.

What would be different if you consciously reflected as a perioperative team, rather than individually?

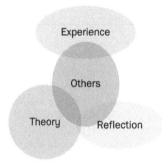

**Figure 8.6** Framework for reflexive learning.
*Source:* adapted from Dyke (2009)

Some of the issues you may have considered will be those already discussed in consequences of reflection. But the nature of your relationship in any group may change and the structure in a group is likely to be less rigid so may result in a deeper and broader analysis of the event. The importance here will be the effect and action on the team as a whole and the professional development of that team.

## Conclusion

This chapter has hopefully provided you with an overview of reflection from the perspective of an ODP. While there is little empirical evidence that reflection can improve patient care (Mann et al., 2009), it has been proven to enhance the process of care, as it is associated with a deeper approach to learning allowing integration with existing knowledge and skills. There is no mystique attached to the process of reflection, it is in its simplest form a process of learning from experience, whether the passive decision making on day-to-day activities such as eating or washing, to the extremes of critical thinking and transforming the very culture of the organization that we are within.

Reflection is not without consequences and challenges to the ODP; it may well trigger emotional responses to be dealt with, find challenges in the relationships of those you work with, have biases and assumptions and even issues of confidentiality and professionalism if undertaken in the public domain of social networking or without forethought.

A range of models is available to guide practitioners though the structured process of reflection; just four have been considered in this chapter. Different models may be needed for every experience and this can be influenced by the event itself, the individual and the context of their role at the time. The development of professional practice will benefit from this type of diversity and it is important to apply models purposefully, selectively and judiciously.

### Key points

- Reflective practice is a key skill for ODPs.
- Reflective practice can be defined as a process to make sense of experiences, events and actions in the practice environment.

- It is a valuable process to enhance professional practice, improve effectiveness and advance life-long learning as an ODP.
- Reflective practice is not without challenges and consequences.
- It enables ODPs to manage their learning and development.
- A toolkit of models to support and guide reflective practice is available to be used appropriately by ODPs.
- Effective reflection can be conducted as an individual, with another, within teams or a mix of both.
- Reflection should not be ritualistic or limited by an algorithmic approach of applying a model or ticking boxes.
- Reflection can allow more critical levels of thinking to emerge and develop.

## References and further reading

Bolton, G. (2010) *Reflective Practice, Writing and Professional Development* (3rd edn). Thousand Oaks, CA: Sage Publications.

Borton, T. (1970) *Reach, Touch and Teach*. London: Hutchinson.

Boud, D., Keogh, R. and Walker, D. (1985) *Reflection: Turning Experience into Learning*. London: Kogan Page.

College of Operating Department Practitioners (CODP) (2011) *Bachelor of Science (Hons) in Operating Department Practice – England, Northern Ireland and Wales, and Bachelor of Science in Operating Department Practice – Scotland, Curriculum Document*. London: CODP.

Conole, G.; Brown, R., Papaefthimiou, M., Alberts, P. and Howell, C. (2010). 'Fostering connectivity and reflection as strategic investment for change', in Ehlers, U.D and Schneckenberg, D. (eds) *Changing Cultures in Higher Education* (pp. 215–32). New York: Springer.

Dewey, J. (1933) *How We Think: A Restatement of the Relation of Reflective Thinking to the Educative Process*. Chicago, IL: Henry Regnery Co.

Dyke, M. (2009) 'An enabling framework for reflexive learning: experiential learning and reflexivity in contemporary modernity', *International Journal of Lifelong Education*, 28 (3): 289–310.

Eraut, M. (1994) *Developing Professional Knowledge and Competence*. Abingdon: Routledge Falmer.

Finlay, L. (2008) 'Reflecting on "reflective practice"', discussion paper 52, Open University, Milton Keynes.

Fitzgerald, M. (1994) 'Theories of reflection for learning, in Palmer, A. and Burns, S. (eds) *Reflective Practice in Nursing*, Oxford, Blackwell Scientific.

Gibbs, G. (1988) *Learning by Doing: A Guide to Teaching and Learning Methods*. Oxford: Oxford Polytechnic.

Greenwood, J. (1993) 'Reflective practice: a critique of the work of Argis and Schön', *Journal of Advanced Nursing*, 19: 1183–187.

Guille, D. and Young, M. (1998) 'Apprenticeship as a conceptual basis for a social theory of learning', *Journal of Vocational Education and Training*, 50 (2): 173.

Hargreaves, J. (2004) 'So how do you feel about that? Assessing reflective practice', *Nurse Education Today*, 24 (3): 196–201.

Health and Care Professions Council (HCPC) (2006) *Standards of Continuing Professional Development*. London: HCPC.

Health and Care Professions Council (HCPC) (2012) *Standards of Conduct, Performance and Ethics*. London: HCPC.

Health and Care Professions Council (HCPC) (2014) *Standards of Proficiency for Operating Department Practitioners*. London: HCPC.

Hobbs, V. (2007) 'Faking it or hating it: can reflective practice be forced?', *Reflective Practice*, 8 (3): 405–17.

Hull, C., Redfern, L. and Shuttleworth, A. (2005) *Profiles and Portfolios: A Guide for Health and Social Care* (2nd edn). New York: Palgrave.

Jasper, M. (1999) 'Nurses' perceptions of the value of written reflection', *Nurse Education Today*, 19 (6): 452–63.

Jasper, M. (2003) *Beginning Reflective Practice*. Cheltenham: Nelson Thornes.

Jay, J.K. and Johnson, K.L. (2002) 'Capturing complexity: a typology of reflective practice for teacher education', *Teaching and Teacher Education*, 18: 73–85.

Johns, C. (1995) 'A philosophical basis for nursing practice', in Johns, C. (ed.) *The Burford NDU Model: Caring in Practice*. Oxford: Blackwell Scientific Publications.

Joyce, P. (2011) 'Professional confidence in Diploma of Higher Education Operating Department Practice students', published thesis, University of Southampton.

Kolb, D. (1984) *Experiential Learning as the Science of Learning and Development*. Upper Saddle River, NJ: Prentice Hall.

Mann, K., Gordon, J. and Macleod, A. (2009) 'Reflection and reflective practice in health professions education: a systematic review', *Advanced Health Science Education*, 2: 1573–677.

Reynolds, M. (1998) 'Reflection and critical reflection in management learning', *Management Learning*, 29 (2), 183–200.

Sandars, J. (2009) 'The use of reflection in medical education: AMEE Guide no 44', *Medical Teacher*, 31: 685–95.

Schön, D. (1983) *The Reflective Practitioner*. New York: Basic Books.

Social Education (2012) *Social Networking Statistics*. Available online at www.statisticbrain.com/social-networking-statistics/

Smyth, J. (1992) 'Teacher's work and the politics of reflection', *American Educational Research Journal*, 29: 267–300.

Wigens, L. (2006) *Expanding Nursing and Health Care Practice*. Cheltenham: Nelson Thornes.

World Health Organization (WHO) (2009) *WHO Surgical Safety Checklist*. London: National Patient Safety Agency.

# 9 Leadership and management for the Operating Department Practitioner

## Michael Donnellon

---

**Key topics**

- Leadership
- Management

- Change theory and management
- Decision making and problem solving

---

## Introduction

Leadership and management have been identified as essential skills for all Operating Department Practitioners (ODPs) and other healthcare staff in order to have the courage to challenge poor practice (The Kings Fund, 2011). This is further supported by a number of national initiates all of which aim to develop leadership within healthcare. New Labour's National Health Service (NHS) Plan (2000) identified that a new Leadership Centre would be established to develop a new generation of managerial and clinical leaders. *High Quality Care for All: NHS Next Stage Review Final Report* (Department of Health (DH), 2008) identified the establishment of a Clinical Management for Quality programme, aimed to equip and support clinicians in leadership and management roles. Currently, the NHS Leadership Academy aims to develop outstanding leadership in health in order to improve a patient's experience of the NHS.

Leadership and management are therefore essential skills for the ODP in order to improve services and patient care. This chapter reviews the theories of leadership and management and provides examples of how the ODP can relate these into their practice. The reader will be encouraged to reflect on leadership and management related issues; there may be no right or wrong answers to these as so often in leadership and management there are so many variables to take into consideration.

## Why is this chapter relevant to ODPs?

ODPs practice in a very complex environment where, to deliver safe, effective care to patients, it is necessary to consider many factors; for example, staffing resources, equipment and the patient's specific needs. It is not only the consideration and synthesis of these factors that is important; however, the ODP also needs to be able to act on this synthesis by making decisions and then leading/managing the action. It is therefore essential that for the delivery of high-quality patient care the ODP develops knowledge and skills of leadership and management. Leadership is also essential for the continued development of the ODP profession for clinical development and also for professional development, by leading our profession through periods of change (College of Operating Department

Practitioners (CODP), 2010) and hence understanding and application of leadership is evident in the Health and Care Professions Council's (HCPC) (2014) *Standards of Proficiency for ODPs*.

## Leadership

All ODPs will demonstrate skills of leadership throughout their careers, starting from their university course; for example, acting as a group lead when undertaking group work through to leading a theatre team or maybe managing a department later in an ODP's career. This therefore demonstrates how leadership underpins all of an ODP's practice, rather than being confined to designated management roles. We have seen therefore that all ODPs demonstrate leadership skills, but what does this really mean?

There are many interpretations of the meaning of leadership. Hersey et al. (2008) define leadership as a process of influencing the behaviour of either an individual or group, regardless of the reason, in an effort to achieve goals in a given situation. Huczynski and Buchanan (2007) view leadership as the process of influencing the activities of an organized group in its efforts towards goal setting and goal achievement. Kotter (2001) expresses leadership as creating vision and strategy, communicating and setting direction, motivating action and aligning people.

### Stop and think

From the definitions of leadership and the suggested examples, consider when have you demonstrated skills of leadership as a student or registered ODP? How well do you think these definitions apply to your role?

### Leadership or management?

It is very common in health and social care to view management and leadership as broadly the same concept with the words being used interchangeably (Martin et al., 2010), and Adair (2008) suggests that there has, and probably always will be, a debate about the differences and overlaps of leadership and management. Current opinion is that that they are different concepts; however, they do overlap considerably and in more recent years, the term 'leader' has been more frequently used to describe someone in a professional or medical role with both management and leadership responsibilities.

In the same way there is conflict between the descriptions of individuals as leaders or managers. McKimm and Philips (2009) cite Bennis and Nanua (1985) who argue that managers are people who do things right and leaders are people who do the right thing. While Barr and Dowding (2009) view that leaders are an essential part of management but the reverse is not true: you do not have to be a manager to be a leader but you do need to be a good leader to be an effective manager.

### NHS Leadership Academy

The NHS Leadership Academy sets out to deliver outstanding leadership in health, in order to improve people's health and their experiences of the NHS. The academy has produced a Leadership Framework (based on the concept of shared or distributed leadership) that is a toolkit that facilitates the leadership development of healthcare professionals including ODPs.

The NHS Leadership Academy (2011) identifies that the Leadership Framework is based on the belief that leadership is not restricted to people who hold designated management and traditional leader roles, but in fact is most successful wherever there is a shared responsibility for the success of the organization, services or care being delivered; this is evident in the operating theatre where a multidisciplinary team share responsibility for the care being delivered to the perioperative patient. The Leadership Framework is comprised of seven domains:

- demonstrating personal qualities;
- working with others;
- managing services;
- improving services;
- setting direction;
- creating the vision;
- delivering the strategy.

The first five domains are referred to as 'core domains' as all staff can contribute to the leadership process by using the behaviours described in the domains. The last two domains relate to those staff that hold designated senior roles and are required to act as leaders in formal hierarchical positions.

In conjunction with the Leadership Framework, the academy has produced a number of self-assessment tools. These tools aim to help ODPs manage their own learning and development by allowing the ODP to reflect on which areas of the Leadership Framework they would like to develop further. The 360° feedback tool involves gaining confidential feedback from line managers and peers and, as a result, gives an individual an insight into other people's perceptions of their leadership abilities and behaviour.

## Approaches to leadership

The concept of leadership can mean different things to different people depending on their various perspectives. Given this, there have been a range of ways identified to classify leadership theories.

### The qualities or traits approach

Popularized in the early part of the twentieth century, this approach (sometimes called Great Man theory) assumes that leaders are born and not made. Leadership consists of certain inherited characteristics or personality traits that distinguish leaders from followers (some are born to lead and others are born to be led). Numerous studies have attempted to identify the qualities and traits found in successful leaders; these include intelligence, motivation, enthusiasm, initiative, courage, vision, high energy levels, physical appearance, speech, self-confidence, popularity, humour and emotional maturity.

Barr and Dowding (2009) suggest that the trait approach has been criticized because it may negate the part that social class, gender and race inequalities play in maintaining the status quo in leadership positions. Martin et al. (2010) highlight that early trait theory was rejected partly because of the implication that if leadership was only as a result of birth, then it was the birthright of some privileged people and not others. Adair (2006) also argues that the list of qualities or traits is very lengthy and that there is a lack of consensus over what are the key or most important qualities of leadership. Furthermore, Adair (2006) highlights that this approach is ill suited to act as a basis for leadership training as instead it encourages a concentration on selection

### The functional or group approach

The functional approach views leadership in terms of how the leader's behaviour affects, and is affected by the group of followers (Mullins, 2011). Kotter (2001) suggests that by concentrating on the functions of the leader, their performance can be improved by training and thus leadership skills can be learned, developed and perfected. Mullins (2011) argues that greater attention can be given to the successful training of leaders and to the means of improving the leaders' performance by concentrating on the functions that will lead to effective performance by the work group.

A contemporary theory on the functional approach to leadership is John Adair's action-centred leadership. A former military lecturer, Adair (2008), argues that a function is what leaders do as opposed to a quality, which is an aspect of what they are. Within action-centred leadership, the effectiveness of the leader is dependent on the leader meeting three areas of need within a work group: task needs, team maintenance needs and individual needs. Ideally, equal attention should be given by the leader to all three areas of need. However, if too much concern is given to any one particular area of need, this can cause an imbalance and can interfere with the effectiveness of the group.

### Leadership as a behavioural category

In this approach, attention is drawn to the kinds of behaviour of people in leadership situations including their leadership style. Leadership style is the way in which the functions of leadership are carried, the way in which the manager typically behaves towards members of the group. The attention given to leadership style is based on the assumption that subordinates are more likely to work effectively for managers who adopt a certain style of leadership than for managers who adopt alternative styles (Mullins, 2011).

There are many ways of describing leadership style such as dictatorial, benevolent and charismatic. However, there are three prominent styles described by writers in the field.

### Authoritarian or autocratic style

In this style, there is a focus on power by the leader and they alone exercise the control and authority over the group. The leader makes decisions alone and will determine policy and work task goals. Expecting obedience, the leader will instigate awards and reprimands.

### Democratic or participative style

A human relations approach is used by leaders favouring this style where the focus of power is more with the group as a whole and teamwork is encouraged. The group members participate in the decision making and will determine policy and goals.

### *Laissez-faire* or genuine style

In this style, the leader uses few established rules deciding rather to pass the focus of power to the group allowing them to work autonomously. However, the leader is available if help is needed. Mullins (2011) highlights that there is sometimes confusion over this style of leadership as the word 'genuine' is to be emphasized as opposed to the leader who avoids the trouble spots and does not want to get involved.

### Stop and think

Are there circumstances within the operating department environment, when the various styles of leadership are more appropriate? For example, during a clinical emergency, which leadership style is most affective?

## Contingency leadership theories

Contingency leadership theory holds the belief that there is no single style of leadership appropriate to all situations, focusing on the flexibility of a leader to choose and adapt an approach in response to different situations – contingencies. One such approach is the path–goal theory developed by the leadership writer Robert House. Path–goal theory is based on the premise that an employee's performance and expectancies are greatly affected by the leader's behaviour as a motivating influence.

Mullins (2011) suggests that in path–goal theory different types of behaviour can be practised by the same person at different times in varying situations and, by using one of the four styles, the manager or leader can influence subordinates' perceptions and motivation and smooth the path to their goals.

## Contemporary leadership theories

In addition to the well-documented leadership theories, the more current approaches are referred to as contemporary theories. Gopee and Galloway (2009) suggest that to an extent, however, these contemporary theories represent further development of the earlier leadership theories and take into account current social, political and organizational factors. Some of the prominent contemporary theories include the following.

### Charismatic

In this approach, leadership is based on the personal qualities of the leader; for example, their charm, persuasiveness, inspiration and self-confidence.

### Servant

The American management researcher, Robert K. Greenleaf, was first to coin the term 'servant leadership' in 1970. In this approach, the servant leader is servant first and leads primarily because of the wish to do good for their followers.

### Transactional

Bass and Riggio (2006) suggest that transactional leadership emphasizes the transaction or exchange that takes place among leaders, colleagues and followers. This exchange is based on the leader discussing with others what is required and specifying the conditions and rewards these others will receive if they fulfil those requirements. Transactional leadership is aimed at maintaining equilibrium or the status quo by performing work according to policy and procedures, maximizing self-interest and personal rewards, and emphasizing interpersonal independence (Sullivan and Decker, 2005).

### Transformational

Bass and Riggio (2006) highlight that transformational leadership involves inspiring followers to commit to a shared vision and goals for an organization or unit, challenging them to be innovative problem solvers, and developing followers' leadership capacity via coaching, mentoring and provision of both challenge and support. Transformational leaders motivate others to do more than they originally intended and often even more than they thought possible. Transformational leaders tend to have more committed and satisfied followers, empowering these followers and paying attention to their individual needs and personal development (Bass and Riggio, 2006). The transformational leadership approach is favoured by the NHS Leadership Academy in that leaders can be developed to 'transform' the behaviours of teams in order to achieve common goals or bring about change.

## Management

Management is a generic term and subject to many interpretations. However, at its most basic, management may be viewed as 'making things happen' (Mullins, 2011). Given this, management can be regarded as:

- taking place within a structured organization setting with prescribed roles (*NHS trust or independent hospital – theatre manager, team leader, principle ODP*);
- directed towards the attainment of aims and objectives *operating theatre efficiency, management of sickness absence, etc.*);
- achieved through the efforts of other people (*the perioperative multidisciplinary team*);
- using systems and procedures (*DH or local trust policies*).

## Theory of management

There have been numerous published theories of management. However, the four main conventional approaches are:

- classical (including scientific management and bureaucratic);
- human relations;
- systems;
- contingency.

### The classical approach

Although one of the earliest management theories, Gopee and Galloway (2009) imply that this approach can still easily be observed in bureaucratic organizations today. In this approach, the emphasis concerns improving the organization structure as a means of increasing efficiency. Attention is given to the division of work where a formal structure is established with regard to exactly who does specific jobs, the clear definition of duties and responsibilities, as well as established rules and procedures for various activities. Emphasis is on a hierarchy of management and formal organizational relationships (Mullins, 2011).

The classical writers included Henri Fayol and Lyndall Urwick. However, it is perhaps Frederick Taylor who is seen as a major contributor due to his writing on scientific management. Taylor believed that in the same way that there is a best machine for each job, so there is a best working method to do a job; that is, breaking jobs into discrete tasks with one best way to perform each task. He also believed that each employee's abilities and limitations should be identified so that the worker could be best matched to the most appropriate job and that financial incentives were a motivator to increase levels of output (Marquis and Huston, 2009).

Rees and Porter (2008) identify that, collectively, the classical theorists viewed workers as rational beings who were capable of working to high levels of efficiency provided they were properly selected, trained, directed, monitored and supported. Although Taylor's work has often been criticized, he has left the legacy of such practices as work study, payment by results and production control.

**Stop and think**

Could the classical approach to management be utilized effectively in order to improve operating theatre efficiency? Make a list of how within a day surgery setting, tasks could be allocated to different grades of staff according to their qualification, educational preparation and competence.

### Human relations approach

During the 1920s, theorists began to pay attention to the social factors at work and to the behaviour of employees within an organization. The human relations era was to emphasize people rather than machines. Leading writers in this approach were Mary Parker Follett and Rensis Likert. Marquis and Huston (2009) identify that Follett believed that managers should have authority with rather than over their employees, thus solutions could be found that satisfied both the employer and employee without having one side dominate the other.

Studies undertaken by Elton Mayo between 1927 and 1932 at the Hawthorne Works of the Western Electric Company near Chicago became a landmark development in the human relations approach. Mayo discovered that if managers paid special attention to workers, productivity was likely to increase and if people worked in groups, especially if the groups were self-selected.

Later developments of the human relations approach included the neo-human relations theories that included the concepts developed by Abraham Maslow (hierarchy of human needs), Frederick Herzberg and Douglas McGregor. McGregor argued that the style of management adopted is a function of the manager's attitudes towards human nature and behaviour at work (Mullins, 2011). He labelled this Theory X and Theory Y. Theory X managers assume that their employees are essentially lazy, need constant supervision and direction, show little responsibility and avoid responsibility. Theory Y managers on the other hand believe that their employees enjoy their work, are self-motivated, ambitious, problem solvers and willing to meet the organizational goals.

Gopee and Galloway (2009) argue that the human relations theory is the most appropriate approach for managing healthcare staff given that the whole ethos of health services is founded on caring and the wellbeing of people. For example, the ODP manager could take into account an individual member of staff's personal and professional development needs:

- Monitoring how a new member of staff is 'settling in' to the operating department.
- Identifying continuing professional development (CPD) opportunities by way of allowing a member of staff to attend workshops, courses or conferences.
- Supporting staff in being creative and encourage them to develop practice improvement projects for the benefit of the department.

### Systems approach

The systems approach attempts to consider and reconcile the advantageous aspects of the classical and human relations approaches. A major contributor to this approach was Ludwig von Bertalanffy. Essentially, this approach recognizes organizations as comprising of a number of systems and subsystems; managers should view organizations both as a whole and as part of a larger environment (Mullins, 2011). Huber (2010) explains that a key principle of the systems theory is that changes in one part of the system affect other parts, creating a ripple within the whole.

**Contingency approach**

The contingency approach stipulates that there is no one optimum state within an organization there-fore the management approach utilized, and its success is dependent or 'contingent' on the nature of tasks with which it is designed to deal with and the nature of environmental influences. Gopee and Galloway (2009) view the contingency approach as comprising the belief that there is no one best and universally applicable management theory as there are a large number of variables and situational factors that have an influence on organizational performance.

## What do managers do?

Management consultancy is big business and the modern management gurus (Michael Porter, Tom Peters, Peter Drucker, Coimbatore Prahalad and Gary Hamel to name but a few) have made small fortunes from their publications and seminars on how managers can 'gain the competitive advan-tage' for their organizations. However, it was Henri Fayol who, in the early twentieth century, first defined managerial activity as the process of forecasting, planning, organizing, commanding, co-ordinating and controlling (Pettinger, 2007).

Mullins (2011) highlights the five basic operations in the work of a manager, as identified by Peter Drucker, which are setting objectives, organizes, motivates and communicates, measures and develops people.

The Canadian academic and management guru, Henry Mintzberg, suggested 10 common roles of a manager that can fall into three categories. Mintzberg (1980) recognized that people who 'manage' have formal authority over the unit they command and this leads to a special position of status within the organization. These roles are given in Table 9.1 with examples relevant for the ODP in a manage-rial position.

**Table 9.1** Ten common roles of the manager

| Category | Role | ODP examples |
| --- | --- | --- |
| Informational | Monitor | Gathers and assesses information related to theatre utilization costs and budgets |
| | Disseminator | Passes on information to staff such as in a team brief, awareness of the MHRA safety warnings, alerts and recalls |
| | Spokesperson | Participate in conferences and meetings outside the organization; for example, with the CODP or the partner higher education institute (HEI) |
| Interpersonal | Figurehead | Represents the department at meetings such as directorate, divisional |
| | Leader | Directs and motivates staff and students by influencing – a role model approach |
| | Liaison | Networks with people within and outside the organization; for example, local education and training boards |
| Decisional | Entrepreneur | Initiates change by or as an example |
| | Disturbance handler | Deals with disputes among staff that arise within the workplace environment |
| | Resource allocator | Decides where to apply resources (both physical i.e. staff, and material i.e. equipment) |
| | Negotiator | Participates in negotiations within team, own organization and external organization; for example human resource department and trade unions |

### Managing people

Although there are many aspects to management, one essential quality of a successful ODP manager is the ability to manage people effectively. Mullins (2011) argues that people generally respond according to the way they are treated. If you give a little, you will invariably get a lot back. This is particularly relevant in the operating department environment given how ODPs need to be so flexible in their working hours in order to cover the unpredictability of operating lists. The majority of staff will respond constructively if treated with consideration and respect. So, how does a manager 'manage people' effectively? Mullins (2011) suggested philosophies are:

- consideration, trust and respect;
- giving of recognition and credit;
- involvement and availability;
- fair and equitable treatment;
- positive action on an individual basis;
- emphasis on end results;
- staff and customer (patient) satisfaction.

### Stop and think

In your work environment do you know a manager that demonstrates any or all of the above qualities? How effective do you think they are?

Have you ever experienced the 'unapproachable manager'? What was so 'unapproachable' about them? Was there an element of 'fear' involved? Were there certain 'good' times when you could approach the manager and 'bad' times when you could not?

Ultimately, which managers get the most out of their staff?

## Management by objectives (MBO)

The MBOs was described by Peter Drucker in 1954 and, as Gopee and Galloway (2009) highlight, directly affects contemporary management in healthcare. In this style of management, the manager aims to 'juxtapose' the organizations' objectives to those of the individual employee and with the employees development needs. During the annual review meeting, the manager and employee jointly identify objectives and targets that are common to both the employee and organization together with a standard and measurement of performance.

Within the NHS, MBO is implemented through the NHS Knowledge and Skills Framework (NHS KSF) and the Development Review Process (DH, 2004) where an ongoing cycle of review, planning, development and evaluation for individuals against the demands of their posts is undertaken. This is a four-stage process that consists of a review of work against agreed objectives and the role, the joint production of a personal development plan, individual learning and development with support from the manager and finally the joint evaluation of learning and development (DH, 2004). This process is continued resulting in the production of a personal development plan (PDP) that identifies the individual's learning and development needs, which are then agreed with the manager and individual.

The main purpose of the development review is to look at the way in which an individual member of staff is developing. The ODP needs to look at this in relation to:

- the duties and responsibilities of their post and current agreed objectives;
- the application of knowledge and skills within the workplace;
- the consequent development needs of the individual member of staff.

---

**Box 9.1 Knowledge and Skills Framework (KSF) related to the ODP**

The KSF defines and describes the knowledge and skills that an ODP needs to apply in their work role. The framework is made up of 'dimensions' that describe different aspects of work. The six dimensions are 'core' to the working of every post within the NHS and were simplified following an independent review of the original dimensions in 2010. The six dimensions are:

1. communication;
2. personal and people development;
3. health, safety and security;
4. service improvement;
5. quality;
6. equality and diversity.

Following the independent review in 2010, a new optional management and leadership dimension was developed for staff in senior roles.

There are a further 24 'specific' dimensions that can be applied to define parts of different posts within the NHS reflecting the post holder's occupational skills. They are grouped into four categories:

1. Health and wellbeing (HWB 1–10)
2. Information and knowledge (IK 1–3)
3. General (G 1–8)
4. Estates and facilities (EF 1–3)

A KSF outline sets out the core and specific dimensions required for a post, setting out a framework for assessment and development of individuals holding that post. Each dimension has four levels called 'indicators'. The higher the level (four is highest), the greater the expectation of the level of knowledge and skills necessary for a post. The dimensions are further described by level descriptors, indicators and references that express each level in more detail.

As you progress in your career as an ODP (on gaining promotion or being employed in an advanced practitioner role) there will be an increase in job responsibilities. As you progress so will the outline for the role. This could include:

- increasing the levels under the core dimensions or requiring more demanding examples of application;
- widening or increasing the number of specific dimensions to include other aspects, particularly managerial or specialist.

*Source:* adapted from NHS Staff Council (2010) *Appraisals and KSF Made Simple: A Practical Guide*

## Change theory and management

Change is inevitable in operating department practice and in particular within the NHS for a number of reasons:

- Change initiated by the election of a new government through implementation of new policy drivers or reforms.
- Change introduced by means of evidence-based practice.
- Change required in meeting the needs and expectations of an ageing population.
- Change due to the impact of technological advances in treating disease.

In his introduction to *Liberating the NHS: Developing the Healthcare Workforce from Design to Delivery* (DH, 2012), the then Secretary of State for Health, commented that today's health workers must be able to cope with ever-changing patient and public needs and adapt quickly to innovation in service models. The recommendations of the Browne Report (Department for Business Innovation and Skills, 2010) brought significant changes in the funding of higher education. For the ODP, therefore, whether in clinical practice, a managerial role or in education, change is unavoidable.

The adoption to new innovations (or change) has been categorized by Rogers and Shoemaker (1972):

- Innovators – individuals who are eager to try new ideas. Have a desire to be hazardous, rash, daring and risky and willing to accept an occasional setback.
- Early adopters – individuals who adopt new ideas early. However, it is the early adopter who other individuals see as the 'man to check with' before using a new idea; they serve as role models for many other members of the team.
- Early majority – individuals who adopt new ideas before the average member of a team, as they may deliberate for some time before completely embracing the new idea.
- Later majority – individuals who will adopt new ideas just after the average member of a team, as they approach with a sceptical and cautious air.
- Laggards – individuals who are the last to adopt an innovation, as their decisions are usually made in terms of what has been done in previous generations. Tend to be suspicious of innovations, innovators and change agents.

Although change can bring its positives, poorly introduced or 'unmanaged' change can be perceived by the employee as fraught with difficulties and threatening. Thornhill et al. (2000) highlight that the implementation of change is likely to be problematic. This is especially likely to be the case in situations where this type of change involves people, and in which personal relationships and emotional responses are predominant. Likewise, Cameron and Green (2009) argue that the consequences of change are significant. For example, who benefits from the changes; the employees or the employer? Who will be the winners and who will be the losers?

Much of the change management literature positions leadership as the key source of energy for change. Carnall (2007) highlights that the process of change can be summarized as being comprised of two elements; namely, leaders and followers. Leaders give signals that changes are needed but without followers no change is possible because leaders cannot do everything. Not all followers will embrace change; neither will all followers resist change.

### Stop and think

What has been the impact of change in your practice?

> Reflect on what changes have been made in your workplace since commencement as an ODP. What 'triggered' these changes? Have some changes been reversed?
>
> Is there an aspect of your practice that you consider would benefit from change?

## Models of change

Documented within management literature are numerous models and theories of organizational change with each model having its own potential benefits or weaknesses? Some that are prominent in the literature include:

- Lewin's 3-Step Model (1947);
- Lippitt's 7-Phase Model of Planned Change (1958);
- McKinsey's 7-S Model (1978);
- Bullock and Batten's 4-Phase Model of Planned Change (1985);
- Cummins and Huse's 8-Phase Model (1989);
- Carnall's Change Management Model (1990);
- William Bridges' Managing the Transition (1991);
- Kotter's 8-Step Process for Leading Change (1995).

Two other models are particularly relevant to healthcare:

- Plan, Do, Study, Act (PDSA) Cycle (1993);
- NHS Change Model (2012).

As with any model or framework, they are tools that help in providing a structured approach to implement change. The ones most relevant to healthcare and in particular the ODP are as follows:

### Lewin's 3-Step Model

Burnes (2004b) highlights that Kurt Lewin's work dominated the theory and practice of change management for over 40 years. However, in the past 20 years his 3-Step Model has attracted some major criticisms. Lewin was a social scientist and had written extensively on a number of approaches to organizational change including field theory, group dynamics and action research. However, it is his work regarding the 3-Step Model that is often cited as his key contribution to organizational change.

Burnes (2004b) cites Lewin (1947) arguing that a successful change project involved three steps:

- Step 1: Unfreezing – Lewin believed that the stability of human behaviour was based on a quasi-stationary equilibrium supported by a complex field of driving and restarting forces. If the equilibrium is destabilized (unfrozen) old behaviour can be discarded and new behaviour successfully adopted.
- Step 2: Moving – movement from a less acceptable to a more acceptable set of behaviours (change)
- Step 3: Refreezing – seeks to stabilize the group at a new quasi-stationary equilibrium in order to ensure new behaviours are relatively safe from regression. In organizational terms, refreezing often requires changes to organizational culture, norms, policies and practices (Burnes, 2004b).

### Bullock and Batten's (1985) 4-Phase Model of Planned Change

Burnes (2004a) highlights that Bullock and Batten (1985) developed an integrated, four-phase model of planned change based on a review and synthesis of over 30 models of planned change.

- Exploration phase – where an organization explores and decides whether it wants to make specific changes in its operations and if so, commits resources to planning the changes. Appoints a consultant/facilitator to assist in the planning.
- Planning phase – understanding of the organization's problems or concerns begins. Information is collected in order to establish a correct diagnosis of the problem. Change goals are established and key decisions makers are persuaded to approve and support changes.
- Action phase – organization implements the changes derived from the planning with movement of the organization from the current state to the desired future state. Evaluation of the implemented activities takes place and results are fed back so that any necessary adjustments or refinements can be made.
- Integration phase – consolidation and stabilizing of the changes established so they become part of the organizations normal everyday operations. Reinforcement of new behaviours through feedback and reward systems undertaken.

## Kotter's 8-Step Process for Leading Change

Acclaimed author and leading authority on leadership and change, John Paul Kotter, introduced his 8-step model in his publication *The 8-Step Process for Leading Change*. Kotter's model first appeared in an article in the March–April 1995 edition of the *Harvard Business Review*. The article listed the mistakes organizations had often made when trying to effect real change and inferred that the 8-stage change framework made sense as a roadmap, helping people talk about transformation, change problems and change strategies (Kotter, 1996).

---

**Box 9.2**

| **Step 1: Establish a Sense of Urgency** | **Step 2: Creating the Guiding** |
|---|---|
| Help the team see the need for change and they will realize the importance of implementing the change without delay | **→ Coalition** <br> Assemble a small group of key team members who can influence positively the change process |
| **Step 4: Communicating the Vision for Buy-in** <br> Communicate the vision to the team ensuring as many members as possible understand and accept the vision | **↓** <br> **Step 3: Developing a Change** <br> **← Vision** <br> Create a vision to help direct the change process |
| **↓** <br> **Step 5: Empowering Broad-based Action** <br> Remove any obstacles to change or the change vision | **Step 6: Generating Short-term** <br> **→ Wins** <br> Plan for achievements that can easily be made visible. Recognize and reward team members who were involved in these achievements |
| **Step 8: Incorporating Changes into the Culture** <br> In simple terms 'make it stick'. Anchor the new approaches into the culture of the team – make these the norm | **↓** <br> **Step 7: Never Letting Up** <br> **← Consolidate** the gains from implementing the change, however, do not be tempted to lose momentum |

*Source:* adapted from www.kotterinternational.com/our-principles/changesteps

### Plan, Do, Study, Act (PDSA) Cycle (1993)

The PDSA Cycle originates from the work undertaken by Deming in 1950 (Moen and Norman, 2010) and is favoured by NHS Improvement, the NHS Institute for Innovation and Improvement, and the American Institute for Healthcare Improvement. The cycle can be used to test an idea by temporarily trailing a change and assessing the impact therefore allowing any refinement of the idea prior to its wider application.

Langley et al. (1994) added three questions to supplement the cycle, entitled 'Model for Improvement', which the PDSA Cycle now forms. These questions consider: what is the aim? Is change an improvement that can be measured? What change can be made to result in an improvement?

The NHS Institute for Innovation and Improvement (2008) have categorized each of the four steps in the cycle:

*Plan*
Define the objective, questions and predictions
Plan to answer the questions (Who? What? Where? When?)
Plan data collection to answer the questions

*Do*
Carry out the plan
Collect the data
Begin analysis of the data

*Study*
Complete the analysis of the data
Compare data to predictions
Summarize what was learned

*Act*
Decide whether the change can be implemented
Plan the next cycle

The Royal College of Anaesthetists (2012) highlight that the simplest form of cyclical examination of practice and change was by using the PDSA methodology to drive small steps of change in practice at a very local level. The NHS Institute for Innovation and Improvement (2008) highlight that the benefits of testing change before implementation should include:

- involves less time, money and risk;
- the process is a powerful tool for learning from both ideas that work and those that do not;
- it is safer and less disruptive for patients and staff;
- because people have been involved in testing and developing the ideas, there is often less resistance.

---

**Stop and think**

*Example of applying the PDSA Cycle and Model of Improvement for the ODP*

NICE Clinical Guideline 65 – *Inadvertent Perioperative Hypothermia: The Management of Perioperative Hypothermia in Adults* (2008) recommends that during the intraoperative phase, intravenous fluids

(500 ml or more) and blood products should be warmed to 37°C using a fluid warming device. Eapen et al. (2009) estimated that if inline fluid warmers were used to implement these guidelines, the cost of the consumables required may be up to £9.45 per patient. In a laboratory evaluation by Eapen et al. (2009), it was found that a less expensive alternative would be the use of fluid that has been prewarmed in a heating cabinet.

A multidisciplinary group (anaesthetists/ODP's/nurses) has been established to evaluate if the temperature of patients who are listed for short duration surgery is adversely affected by the use of delivering prewarmed intravenous fluid. The group intend to use a PDSA Cycle to test this approach. Consider how the PDSA Cycle can be employed to undertake the evaluation.

## NHS Change Model (2012)

The NHS Change Model has been created to support the NHS to adopt a shared approach to leading change and transformation. The model has been developed by senior leaders, clinicians, commissioners, providers and improvement activists who wanted to become involved in building the energy for change across the NHS by adopting a systematic and sustainable approach to improving quality (NHS, 2012).

The model brings together collective improvement knowledge and experience from across the NHS into the following eight key components:

- speed of innovation;
- improvement methodology;
- rigorous delivery;
- transparent measurement;
- system drivers;
- engagement to mobilize;
- leadership for change.

## Resistance to change

Despite the potential positive outcomes, change is often resisted at both individual and organization level (Mullins, 2011). Carnall (2007) suggests that change is difficult as one must inevitably deal with people issues and an uncertain future. Tyler (2007) identified that a common problem associated with change is that it may create unintended consequences.

Mabey and Salaman (1995), cited in Thornhill et al. (2000), consider a number of perceptions about the management of change that will affect reactions to it. Among these factors is whether change is perceived as 'deviant or normal' and 'threatening or desirable'. Change judged as deviant can be perceived to be imposed and outside prevailing cultural norms therefore likely to generate resistance at various levels. Change seen as threatening is also likely to meet resistance and will require careful implementation to overcome the fear associated with this perception.

Resistance to change can take two forms; overt where people are open about why they are against the change (preferable form) or covert where individuals or groups try to sabotage the change secretly. This covert form is much more damaging and harder to deal with (Marquis and Huston, 2009).

Mullins (2011) identifies common reasons for individual resistance to change. These reasons are given in Table 9.2 with examples of how an ODP could possibly be affected.

**Table 9.2** Reasons for resistance to change

| Reason | Example | ODP example |
|---|---|---|
| Selective perception | People can have a biased view of a particular situation | • Role boundaries (e.g. anaesthesia, surgical, post-anaesthetic care) |
| Habit | Habits serve as a means of comfort and security | • Regular shift patterns<br>• Allocation to a regular operating theatre<br>• Regular car parking spot! |
| Inconvenience or loss of freedom | Change could make life more difficult | • Changes to regular shift patterns<br>• Introduction of some method of 'clocking-on/ clocking-off system |
| Economic implications | Either directly or indirectly a reduction in pay or other rewards or a threat to their job security | • Reduction in amount of 'on-call' or extra duty payments<br>• Pay freeze<br>• Review of job role or pay banding |
| Security in the past | When faced with new or unfamiliar ideas or methods, people may reflect on a sense of security in the past | • Change due to the introduction of a new policy or practice<br>• Change due to the introduction of new equipment<br>• Change due to working with a new team |
| Fear of the unknown | Changes in work organization may present a degree of uncertainty leading to anxiety or fear | • Restructuring of directorate or department<br>• Amalgamation of two NHS Trust |

## Overcoming resistance to change

Carnall (2007) suggests that much of what is referred to as 'resistance to change' is 'resistance to uncertainty' therefore the resistance derives from how the process is handled and less so of what is being changed. If people understand what is to be achieved, why, how and by whom, this will contribute to the understanding and how this will impact on what it means to them.

In a prominent article on the subject, Kotter and Schlesinger (1979) argued that many managers underestimated not only the variety of ways people could react to change, but also the ways in which managers could positively influence specific individuals or groups during change. Kotter and Schlesinger (1979) set out the following six changes approaches to deal with the resistance of change:

## Education and communication

One of the most common ways to overcome resistance to change is to educate people about it beforehand. Communication of ideas helps people see the need for and the logic of change and once persuaded people will often help with the implementation of the change.

### Participation and involvement

If the initiators involve the potential resistors in some aspect of the design and implementation of the change, they can often forestall resistance. With a participative change effort, the initiators listen to the people the change involves and use their advice.

### Facilitation and support

This process might include providing training in new skills, or simply listening and providing emotional support. Facilitation and support are most helpful when fear and anxiety lie at the heart of resistance.

### Negotiation and agreement

Offering incentives to active or potential resistors is a way of dealing with resistance. Negotiation is particularly appropriate when it is clear that someone is going to lose out as a result of change and yet their power to resist is significant.

### Manipulation and co-option

Co-opting an individual usually involves giving them a desirable role in the design or implementation of the change. Co-opting a group involves giving one of its leaders, or someone it respects, a key role in the design or implementation of change.

### Explicit and implicit coercion

In this approach, people are forced to accept a change by being explicitly or implicitly threatened (i.e. loss of promotion possibilities), or by being transferred to another department within the organization or by being dismissed.

### Acceptance of change

Kirkpatrick (1993) identified nine reasons why people either accept or welcome change:

- Expect more favourable working conditions or an increase in income and status.
- Expect more opportunities for growth, recognition and promotion.
- Think the change will provide new challenges and lessen boredom.
- Think the change is needed and the timing is right.
- Like or respect the person or department that introduced the change.
- Like the way the change was introduced.
- Contributed input to the change.
- Have positive feelings about the organization or their jobs.
- Have been positively influenced by their peers or leaders of their peer groups.

### Stop and think

Joe, an experienced theatre practitioner has worked on a day surgery operating theatre for six years. Sessions times on this operating theatre are currently Monday to Friday only; however, the theatre manager wishes to introduce a rotational system that would cover weekends which all staff will require to participate in. Joe objects to the manager's suggestion quoting 'custom and practice'.

Does Joe have a valid point? If forced to comply with the new system, could Joe claim grievance? If Joe does not comply, could this be viewed as him being deliberately obstructive? What could be considered a 'reasonable comprise' in Joe's situation?

## Decision making and problem solving

Earlier in this chapter, it has been identified that decision making is part of the manager's role. Huber (2010) suggests decision making is the essence of leadership and management while Marquis and Huston (2009) highlight that decision making is often thought to be synonymous with management and is one of the criteria of which management expertise is judged.

Although decision making and problem solving appear similar, they are not synonymous. Decision making may or may not involve a problem, but it does involve selecting one of several alternatives, each of which may be appropriate under the circumstances. Problem solving however involves diagnosing a problem and solving it, which may or may not entail deciding on the correct solution (Sullivan and Decker, 2009).

Table 9.3 identifies activities encountered by the ODP that require either the making of a decision, a problem to be solved or both.

**Table 9.3** ODP decision making and problem solving

| Activity | Decision making or problem solving |
| --- | --- |
| During check-in procedure, patient informs you that they had a drink one hour previously | Decision making |
| During checking of anaesthetic machine, fault found on ventilator | Decision making and problem solving |
| During needle, swab and instrument count, swab missing | Decision making and problem solving |
| Member of staff phones in sick | Problem solving |
| Which staff to send on a transfer | Decision making |
| A student complains of being unfairly treated by a mentor | Problem solving |

### Decision making

It can be seen from Table 9.3 that some of the decisions encountered by the ODP can be big or small/ complex or straightforward. *Routine decisions* are often made by use of policies and procedures. *Adaptive decisions* are required to be made when the problem and alternative solutions are somewhat unusual and only partially understood. The decision made is by adapting a decision made in a previous similar situation. *Innovative decisions* are made when the problem is unusual, unclear or unprecedented, requiring creative or novel solutions to be made.

Stott (1992), cited in Barr and Dowding (2009), also identified that not all decisions are of equal importance in that when making decisions, some will involve either greater or lesser time commitment, some will require additional skills, some will involve many people and some will require a greater or lesser amount of resources.

- *Standard decisions* – those made on a daily basis and tend to be repetitive. Solutions are usually found by policies or procedures. An example of this would be when reporting a fault on a piece of equipment to the electro-biomedical engineering (EBME) department.
- *Crisis decisions* – these are made in unexpected situations and require an immediate response with little time to negotiate and plan with others. An example of this would be when being notified that a patient has a ruptured aortic aneurysm and requires immediate surgery.
- *Deep decisions* – those made when there is a requirement for more intense planning, reflection and consideration. An example of this would be when considering building an additional operating theatre or part of the change management process.

## Decision-making process

There are a number of approaches to the decision-making process. The *political decision-making model* is the process in which the particular interests and objectives of powerful stakeholders influence the decisions made by others; for example, clinical commissioning groups, local education and training boards, and regulatory bodies

The *rational decision-making model* is based on the making of logical, well-grounded rational choices that maximize the achievement of objectives. Sullivan and Decker (2009) describe the *descriptive rationality model* that was developed by Simon in 1995. This model emphasizes the limitations of the rationality of the decision maker and the situation. It recognizes three ways in which decision makers depart from the rational decision-making model:

- The decision maker's search for possible objectives or alternative solutions is limited because of time, energy or money.
- People frequently lack adequate information about problems and cannot control the conditions under which they operate.
- Individuals often use a strategy that is not ideal but is good enough under the circumstances to meet the minimum standards of acceptance.

The decision-making process begins when a gap exists between what is actually happening and what should be happening, and it ends with action that will narrow or close this gap (Sullivan and Decker, 2009). The 7-Step Decision-making Model breaks the decision making into individual components as outlined in Box 9.3.

---

### Box 9.3 The 7-Step Decision-making Model

1. Identify the purpose
2. Set the criteria
3. Weigh the criteria
4. Seek alternatives
5. Test alternatives
6. Troubleshoot
7. Evaluate the action

(Sullivan and Decker, 2009)

---

When faced with a routine or standard decision, local policies and procedures can usually produce a satisfactory result within a short period of time. For those adaptive decisions, there are a number of decision-making techniques or tools that can assist in the problem analysis in order to compare outcomes of alternative solutions. These include simple flow charts, decision trees, fishbone diagrams, problem continuums, cause-and-effect diagrams and consequence tables.

A decision tree is a graphic model that visually displays the options, outcomes and risks to be anticipated (Figure 9.1). Normally, decision trees start at the left identifying the question or problem and flow to the right identifying the possible options, consequences and costs that become branch nodes. For example, a decision tree may start with the question 'How to reduce waiting lists?'

Clancy (2003) highlights that there is a tendency for managers to unconsciously favour first impressions when making decisions and once established, a second tendency labelled 'confirmation bias' can follow. A confirmation bias consists of the tendency to affirm one's initial impression and preferences as other alternatives are evaluated. Even the use of decision-making tools therefore will not guarantee a successful decision.

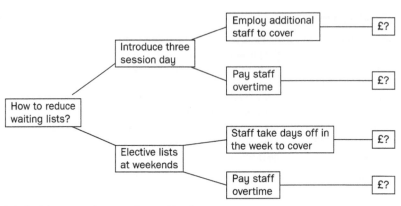

**Figure 9.1** Decision tree on how to reduce waiting list.

## Problem solving

Some problems are self-solving, that is, if the problem runs a natural cause, the problem is solved by those personally involved without any intervention by the manager. However, this can carry a fair amount of risk as the problem can manifest and when intervention is required, the manager may now face a far more complex situation to deal with.

As with decision making, there are a variety of methods to solve problems. The *trial and error* method is when one solution is applied after another until the problem is solved or appears to be improving. Huber (2010) infers that managers, who often use trial and error as the usual strategy for decision making, are seen as ineffective and perceived as poor problem solvers. *Experimentation* is more rigorous than trial and error and can involve the use of pilot projects and trials. An example of this could be the introduction of an on-call system to replace permanent night staff. After a period of time, data can be collected and analysed to determine whether the project has been effective in solving the problem

Problem-solving models also exist and one of the most widely used is the 7-Step Problem-solving Process:

- Define the problem – does the problem really exist? Is there an existing policy or protocol that could alleviate the problem?
- Gather the information – it is important to gather as much accurate information as possible about the problem from a variety of sources in order that informed decisions can be made.
- Analyse the information – list and categorize the information
- Develop solutions – there could be a number of alternative solutions therefore it is important to not only consider the simple solutions but to consider the more complex ones also. Solutions to long-standing problems may have been suggested previously therefore take these into account. Past experience may not supply the answer but can aid in the problem-solving process.
- Make decision – after reviewing all of the information and identifying possible solutions, select the one that is most applicable and feasible in order to solve the problem.
- Implement the decision – implement the preferred solution. There is always the risk of the unintended consequences materializing.
- Evaluate the solution – after the solution has been implemented, review the plan and compare the results with what was originally the ideal solution.

Marquis and Huston (2009) argue that although this is an effective model, its weakness lies in the amount of time needed for proper implementation.

**Stop and think**

In your role as practice educator, Rachel a Year 1 student ODP approaches you with concerns about her mentor. Rachel implies that her mentor is not permitting her the opportunity to undertake certain skills. When Rachel's mentor does allocate a task, she feels the mentor is always critical of her performance, in Rachel's words, 'picks me up for the slightest thing'. On previous placements, Rachel had developed good relationships with other mentors and had demonstrated competence in tasks allocated. You decide to discuss the issue with the mentor who informs you that in their opinion, Rachel had displayed little enthusiasm on placement, appeared more concerned about completing her theoretical assignments from university and at times her professional approach to other members of the multidisciplinary team was questionable.

The dilemma for the practice educator – is this just a class of personalities or is an intervention required? Could an intervention deteriorate the situation? Remember, there are *three* sides to every story!

### Group problem solving

The advantage of groups is that collectively, groups have greater knowledge and experience than any single member and may produce more solutions or approaches to solve a problem. Leadership of the group is important and this will be influenced by the leaders style be it autocratic, democratic or *laissez-faire*.

Together, groups can generate more complete, accurate and less biased information than one person (Sullivan and Decker, 2009). However, Barr and Dowding (2009) argue that some caution must be taken in that individuals within groups may conform to the majority decision due to group pressure, or feeling uncomfortable as they could be perceived as the outsider.

## Conclusion

This chapter has examined leadership and management theories and styles, how change can be managed and the complexities of decision making and problem solving. Given the ever-increasing demands of healthcare services, now more than ever does the NHS require effective leaders. A key recommendation of the Public Enquiry into the Mid Staffordshire NHS Foundation Trust (Francis, 2013) identified the particular importance of leaders setting examples of applying the common culture and values of the NHS.

At the beginning of this chapter, it was stated that leadership and management are essential skills for the ODP in order to improve services and care. As more and more ODPs are employed in managerial and advance practitioner roles, their leadership and management skills will require developing. Knowledge of these key skills require inclusion in any pre-registration healthcare programme as the students of today are the leaders of tomorrow.

**Key points**

- Leadership is a fundamental skill for the ODP and therefore it is important to understand the theory that underpins this.
- Management theories that relate to the ODP.
- Change theory and management is essential for ODPs who work within an environment that is continually changing.

- Decision making and problem solving are key aspects of the ODP's role and there are a variety of approaches to support these processes.

## References and further reading

Adair, J. (2006) *Effective Leadership Development*. London: Chartered Institute of Personnel and Development.

Adair, J. (2008) *The Best of Adair on Leadership and Management*. London: Thorogood Publishing.

Barr, J. and Dowding, L. (2009) *Leadership in Healthcare*. London: Sage Publications.

Bass, B.M. and Riggio, R.E. (2006) *Transformational Leadership* (2nd edn). Mahwah, NJ: Lawrence Erlbaum Associates.

Burnes, B. (2004a) *Managing Change: A Strategic Approach to Organisational Development*. Harlow: Financial Times Prentice Hall.

Burnes, B. (2004b) 'Kurt Lewin and the planned approach to change', *Journal of Management Studies*, 41 (6): 977–1002.

Cameron, E. and Green, M. (2009) *Making Sense of Change Management* (2nd edn). London: Kogan Page.

Carnall, C.A. (2007) *Managing Change in Organisations* (5th edn). Harlow: Financial Times Prentice Hall.

Clancy, T.R. (2003) 'The art of decision making', *Journal of Nursing Administration*, 33 (6): 343–49.

College of Operating Department Practitioners (CODP) (2010) 'Framing the future role and function of Operating Department Practitioners', discussion paper. London: CODP.

Department for Business Innovation and Skills (2010) *The Browne Report: Securing a Sustainable Future for Higher Education. An Independent Review of Higher Education Funding and Student Finance*. London: Department for Business Innovation and Skills.

Department of Health (DH) (2000) *The NHS Plan: A Plan for Investment, A Plan for Reform*. London: DH.

Department of Health (DH) (2004) *The NHS Knowledge and Skills Framework (NHS KSF) and the Development Review Process*. London: DH.

Department of Health (DH) (2008) *High Quality Care for All: NHS Next Stage Review Final Report*. London: DH.

Department of Health (DH) (2012) *Liberating the NHS: Developing the Healthcare Workforce from Design to Delivery*. London: DH.

Department of Health (DH) and Social Security (DHSS) (1983) *The Griffiths Report on the National Health Service*. London: DHSS.

Eapen, G., Andrzejowski, J. and Turnbull, D. (2009) 'A laboratory evaluation of the heat generating capacity of prewarmed fluid compared with two commercial in-line fluid warming devices', *Anaesthesia*, 64 (7): 806.

Ellis, P. and Bach, S. (2011). *Leadership, Management and Team Working in Nursing*. London: Sage Publications.

Francis, R. (2013) *The Report of the Mid Staffordshire NHS Foundation Trust Public Enquiry*. London: The Stationery Office.

Gopee, N. and Galloway, J. (2009) *Leadership and Management in Healthcare*. London: Sage Publications.

Health and Care Professions Council (HCPC) (2014) *Standards of Proficiency Operating Department Practitioners*. London: HCPC.

Hersey, P., Blanchard, K.H. and Johnson, D.E. (2008) *Management of Organisational Behaviour; Leading Human Resources* (9th edn). Upper Saddle River, NJ: Prentice Hall.

House, R.J. (1996) 'Path-goal theory of leadership: lessons, legacy, and a reformulated theory', *Leadership Quality*, 7 (3): 323-52.

Huber, D. (2010) *Leadership and Nursing Care Management* (4th edn). Philadelphia, PA: Saunders.

Huczynski, A. and Buchanan, D.D. (2010) *Organisational Behaviour: An Introductory Text*. Harlow: Financial Times Prentice Hall.

Kanter, R.M. (1985) 'Managing the human side of change', *Management Review*, 74 (4): 52–57.

Kirkpatrick, D.L. (1993) 'Riding the winds of change', *Training and Development*, 47 (2): 28–32.

Klein, R. (1989) *The Politics of the N.H.S.* Harlow: Longman Group Ltd.

Kotter, J.P. (1996) *Leading Change*. Boston, MA: Harvard Business School.

Kotter, J.P. (2001) 'What leaders really do', *Harvard Business Review The Magazine*, pp. 85–98.

Kotter, J.P. and Schlesinger, L.A. (1979) 'Choosing strategies for change', *Harvard Business Review*, 57 (2): 106–14.

Kotter, P. (2012) *The 8 Step Process for Leading Change*. Available online at http://www.kotterinternational.com/our-principles/changesteps

Langley, G., Nolan, K. and Nolan, T. (1994) 'The foundation of improvement', *Quality Progress*, 27 (6): 81–87.

Marquis, B.L. and Huston, C.J. (2009) *Leadership Roles and Management Functions in Nursing: Theory and Application* (6th edn). Philadelphia, PA: Wolters Kluwer/Lippincott Williams and Williams.

Martin, V., Charlesworth, J. and Henderson, E. (2010) *Managing in Health and Social Care* (2nd edn). London: Routledge.

McKimm, J. and Philips, K. (2009) *Leadership and Management in Integrated Services*. Exeter: Learning matters Ltd.

Mintzberg, H. (1980) *The Nature of Managerial Work*. Englewood Cliffs, NJ: Prentice Hall.

Moen, R.D. and Norman, C.L. (2010) 'Circling back: clearing the myths about the Deming cycle and seeing how it keeps evolving quality progress', *Quality Progress*, 43 (11): 22–28.

Mullins, L.J. (2011) *Essentials of Organisational Behaviour* (3rd edn). Harlow: Pearson Education Ltd.

National Health Service (NHS) Leadership Academy (2011) *Leadership Framework*. Coventry: National Health Service (NHS) Institute for Innovation.

National Health Service (NHS) (2012) *NHS Change Model*. Available online at http://www.changemodel.nhs.uk/pg/dashboard

National Health Service (NHS) Staff Council (2012) *Appraisals and KSF Made Simple – A Practical Guide*. London: NHS Employers.

National Institute of Health and Clinical Excellence (NICE) (2008) NICE Clinical Guideline 65 – *Inadvertent Perioperative Hypothermia: The Management of Perioperative Hypothermia in Adults*. London: NICE

Pettinger, R. (2007) *Introduction to Management*. Basingstoke: Palgrave Macmillan.

Rees, W.D. and Porter, C. (2008) *Skills of Management* (6th edn). London: South-Western Cengage Learning.

Rogers, E.M. and Shoemaker, F.F (1972) *Communications of Innovations: A Cross-cultural Approach* (2nd edn). New York: Free Press.

Royal College of Anaesthetists (2012) *Raising the Standard: A Compendium of Audit Recipes for Continuous Quality Improvement in Anaesthesia*. London: Royal College of Anaesthetists.

Sullivan, E.J. and Decker, P.J. (2009) *Effective Leadership and Management in Nursing* (7th edn). Upper Saddle River, NJ: Prentice Hall.

The Kings Fund (2011) *The Future of Leadership and Management in the NHS: No More Heroes*. London: The Kings Fund.

Thornhill, A., Lewis, P., Millmore, M. and Saunders, M. (2000) *Managing Change: A Human Resource Strategy Approach*. London: Prentice Hall.

Tyler, S. (2007) *The Manager's Good Study Guide* (3rd edn). Maidenhead: Open University Press.

# Professional practice for Operating Department Practitioners

## *Stephen Wordsworth*

---

**Key topics**

- What is meant by the term 'professional practice' and what determines who the professions are

- Professional values, judgement, decision making and clinical reasoning – as professional key professional qualities.

- Legal, professional and regulatory accountability and the role of the Health Care and Professions Council (HCPC) in maintaining and supporting clinical conduct and competence

- Scope of practice and developing advanced practice

---

## Introduction

This chapter outlines the concepts and meaning of professional practice from a range of perspectives and viewpoints. It looks at the issues of definition and explores who the 'professions' are and what is understood by the term 'professionalism' in the healthcare setting. It takes a theoretical perspective and refers to some key research to explore why definitions of a profession and professionalism are changing. These address a number of contemporary themes that relate to the Operating Department Practitioner (ODP) such as professional values and beliefs, professional judgement and decision making, as well as clinical reasoning as a key professional competence.

This chapter explores principles of professionalism including legal and regulatory accountability, along with an exploration of the role and function of the HCPC. There are key interrelated concepts such as autonomy, delegation and supervision that will be considered in relation to current debates around advanced practice and a greater appreciation of topics such as scope of practice, advanced practice, misconduct and performance and fitness to practice. The chapter concludes by summarizing what has emerged and the issues that still need to be addressed within the contemporary context of the ODPs' professional practice.

## Why is this relevant?

Most ODPs probably describe themselves as professionals in conversations or debates with colleagues in the perioperative environment. This is certainly the case at university were students are taught the principles of professionalism during their studies. ODPs might even use the term to describe and explain what their job entails to family and friends. The extent, however, to whether this is largely rhetorical, is still not clear. Saying that 'I am a professional', rather than acting according to the principles of professionalism, are potentially two different things. As a starting point it might be useful to consider which occupational groups constitute being classed as a profession and why. This might seem obvious but I should warn you that the terms 'profession' and 'professional', and what it means to act in a professional manner, are contested because they are open to interpretation and therefore disagreement. There is always a danger that the idea of being a professional is of symbolical importance rather than becoming an embedded feature of what it means to practise as an ODP.

ODPs have been subject to statutory regulation for over 10 years, but has their professionalism and their professional practice changed? After all the status that comes with being recognized as a statutory profession should not be mistaken for the perceived benefits of increased salaries or better working conditions, over improvements in the care of the surgical patient. Similarly, ODPs may also aspire to the autonomy afforded to other professional groups while simultaneously not realizing that as a profession, this brings with it commitments to accountability, both for their actions and omissions.

## Stop and think

Why do you think that ODPs can justify their status as a profession?

## What is a profession: the problem with definition?

In order to address whether this critique may be true, it is necessary to begin to consider what profession means. From a sociological perspective, that is, from a viewpoint of how society is organized and experienced, Friedson (1994: 13) tells us that:

Until recently, most sociologists have been inclined to see professions as honoured servants of public need, conceiving of them as occupations especially distinguished by their orientation to serving the needs of the public through the schooled application of their unusual esoteric knowledge and complex skill.

To what extent does this definition still ring true? From an economic perspective, training more healthcare professionals is costly, so why go to the expense when healthcare assistants (HCAs) or assistant practitioners (APs) could do the job? From the perspective of public need, politicians have been increasingly critical of the power and privilege, particularly, of the medical profession, in holding the government to ransom over healthcare reforms (Elston, 1991). Health policy makers though constantly seem to want to 'blur existing professional boundaries', which they see as narrow and restrictive, and leads to the ghettoization of skills and knowledge (Curry and Suhomlinova, 2006). So in many ways power and specialist skills in the hands of a few no longer fits the public need.

Based on Friedson's (1994) definition, the idea of a relatively small number of prestigious occupations would in the past have singled them out largely on the basis of their access to a university education. Historically, this select group would have included those wanting to practise in medicine, the law or, in earlier times, the priesthood. However, as a result of the democratization and expansion of higher education (HE) that has taken place, many new occupational groups now complete a HE qualification (Reay et al., 2005). This form of credentialism of profession qualifications now makes it possible to argue that ODPs, as well as other allied health professions and nurses, along with a plethora of other occupational groups such as social workers, teachers, accountants and architects, now meet the conditions once reserved for elite social occupations. Indeed, since the adoption of the College of Operating Department Practitioners (CODP) (formally AODP) initial HE curriculum in

2001, ODPs now qualify with a university qualification; which meets our own professional standards and reflects the specialist nature of our knowledge and practice. Sometimes this so-called 'body of knowledge', if not esoteric, is at least common to all ODPs, and indeed can be shared in part with other theatre practitioners. So while it is possible to make a case that suggests ODPs now meet established criteria, inevitably there are some who would argue that true professions exist purely as a result of the status they hold in society.

A useful way of exploring how status and qualifications are important to the development of the professions is through the work of the sociologist Pierre Bourdieu. He argues that maintaining profession status is possible because of the capital that the professions confer upon their members. For Bourdieu (1984) capital is a complex interplay of cultural and social advantages that develop over a period of time. Bourdieu (2006) also suggested that 'capital begets capital', so to join the professions you need to have the benefits of social advantage and educational ability, and when you eventually qualify your capital increases further.

### Theorizing the professions

Bourdieu predicts that some professions (or social group) are able to impose their status more than others. He calls this process 'symbolic violence' or the domination of one occupation over another; consider how doctors and nurses dominate the field of healthcare. The theory of capital can also be useful to explain the status and historic differences between ODPs and perioperative nurses and how such 'occupational boundary disputes' (Timmons and Tanner, 2004: 645) will remain while ODPs are still engaged in gaining capital and therefore professional recognition.

Karl Marx felt that capital was based on the relative value of professional skills and knowledge to the economy and to the state. Macdonald's (1995: 23) theoretical review identifies how Marxist theory suggests that the professions are inextricably linked to economic production and the wealth of the nation. Therefore the true value of the ODP is not in the role itself, but in contribution to the healthcare economy and to the preservation of the state-run National Health Service (NHS). Max Weber (1978) makes the case that professional qualifications define what is now called the middle classes, and therefore the professions are important to define social class. Latterly Diane Reay and colleagues (2005) have written extensively on how access to university qualifications has led to the development of a number of new professions, particularly in healthcare. Over time such changes in social status should help cement the ODP's professional status much as Weber has suggested.

Theories of the professions perhaps culminate in the work of Foucault (1977) as he states that there is a 'genealogy' between the power of the state and legal systems to hold others to account. In exchange for becoming part of the established order, some occupations receive a form of state patronage. This same process has ultimately led to the regulation for ODPs, and was initially granted when the NHS Executive (2000) issued guidance that basically handed legitimacy to the College of Operating Department Practitioners (CODP), by insisting that all ODPs working in the NHS must submit to a voluntary scheme of registration maintained by the CODP. However, the extent of this legitimization is potentially challenged by Timmons (2011) who argues that professionalization, in the context of ODP, comes at a price:

For many groups, the state is now so comprehensively dominant in the process of professionalization that it can effectively dictate professional status on its own terms. Many of the advantages that accrued to professions that developed historically will not be available to groups that professionalize under this new regime.

Timmons argues that the endorsement of new health professions such as that recently extended to ODP is, in reality, limited to regulation, which could be seen as restrictive, intrusive and even anti-democratic.

From a different perspective the HCPC (2011: 4) cogently recognize the changing context of professionalism:

Professions which are newly 'professionalised' may find it harder to gain this support and recognition than more established ones. The context specific nature of professionalism means that further work in this area should address the development of professionalism as a dynamic judgment rather than a discrete skill set.

Viewing professionalism in this way opens up the possibility to identify and explore a range of attributes not identified in elitist, hierarchical or patriarchal (Witz, 1992) models of the professions.

## New debates around professionalism

So far, we have seen how traditional definitions provide a rather 'static' construction of the notion of what is a profession. This stems from status and is largely based around skills and competence. A number of commentators have suggested that this is still the case in the field medical education (see Cruess and Cruess, 2006; Stern, 2006). However, it is perhaps now time to move away from such definitions, partly because consensus has not been achieved. Furthermore, static definitions also ignore the fact that the spotlight is not now necessarily on the skills of individuals but on their attitudes, values and behaviours; in short, on their *professionalism*. In a major study on the subject the HCPC (2011: 5) suggest that:

'Professionalism' is under increasing scrutiny across the health and social care professions, with many of the issues that emerge later in people's careers being linked to a broad range of behaviours distinct from their technical ability.

The HCPC study commissioned research that undertook to gather the views and opinions of a range of professions that they regulate. This took into account the views of students, qualified practitioners and managers alike. From the study the data was categorized in such a way to conceptualize what constitutes professionalism from a number of emerging perspectives. This study identified several key dimensions of professionalism that are now explained in turn.

### Professionalism as a holistic concept

The first category identified professionalism as a whole, rather than a discrete set of characteristics. The researchers found that participants talked in universal terms, as an 'all-encompassing concept ("everything you do"), an overall way of being that comprises a range of attitudes and behaviours'. The report also highlights how some respondents considered their role reflexively, or how they would like to be treated themselves if they were the patient.

Some recent research into career choice in the Allied Health Professions also found that student responses closely matched the holistic concept of the professional. Students articulated a desire 'to help people who will need care and support' and 'to help improve the quality of people's lives' (Wordsworth, 2011).

### Professionalism as good clinical care

The second characteristic identified in the HCPC study defines professionalism as the need to demonstrate technical skills and competence. Participants in their study stressed the importance of an ongoing 'ability to do the job'. However, the essence of professional practice was also wrapped up in the ability of practitioners to know and understand their limitations, and seek out ways to keep their skills up to date. Again, in the research study on student choice, some students felt more useful and trusted, and indeed 'part of the team' the more technically competent they became (Wordsworth,

2011). The HCPC (2011) study also highlights the importance of maintaining patient trust and confidence as a key characteristic of professionalism and their accountability. Reflection on their practice and keeping up to date are viewed as complementary features of good clinical care.

**Stop and think**

What personal qualities and professional skills do you have that are necessary for patients to have trust in your ability to provide effective and compassionate clinical care?

### Professionalism as an expression of self

The HCPC (2011) study found that the notion of professionalism was somehow intrinsically linked to the expression of self. In the minds of practitioners and educators alike, being a professional was a deeply held 'core belief' that defines their actions and thoughts, a quality that underpins their practice through their own pre-existing meta-qualities. Importantly the (HCPC, 2011: 15) study demonstrates how being a professional 'is a way of life'. Therefore, there is an expectation that professionalism and the qualities necessary to maintain this extend to all aspects of their lives, including those beyond work. Rather than suggesting the innateness of professionalism, professionalism 'becomes part of the professional'.

Inevitably this blurring of boundaries leads to uncertainty as to how far one's personal life should be influenced by the need to remain professional at all times. Other respondents in the HCPC (2011: 15) study were less keen to be 'defined by the job' and were concerned by the blurring of their 'professional and private self'. This has important consequences for their conduct and the role of the regulator in holding a practitioner to account for their lack of professionalism. One particular area of concern is the inappropriate use of social media, and is cited in a growing number of student fitness to practice cases. The use of social media can raise issues of misconduct and this can typically result in breaches of confidence and trust, defamation, as well as bringing the profession or institution into disrepute. Recent changes to the HCPC's *Standards of Education and Training* (SETs) (point 3.16) now reflect the fact that healthcare education programmes must have in place systems for addressing concerns about a student's behavior (HCPC, 2012d).

**Stop and think**

Where you could find guidance on the use of social media and fitness to practise procedures, then consider how your personal life could impact upon you and your professional life?

Misuse of social media suggests that some students and practitioners lack a sense of personal insight that is not learned as part of the role. Participants in the HCPC (2011) study suggested that these qualities were gained through their social and cultural upbringing and from their family experiences, often with key people such as their parents acting as role models. That said clinical role models from their training were also important to the way that students ultimately expressed their own sense of professionalism.

Other professional attributes identified in the HCPC (2011) study centred on having the right attitude to study, enthusiasm for the job and a commitment towards positive relationships with colleagues and patients. Not surprisingly the importance of good communication surfaced as did:

- politeness;
- trustworthiness and honesty;
- acting calmly and confidently;
- being personable.

The final noteworthy area of professionalism from the HCPC (2011) study involved the practitioner's appearance. Findings suggest that wearing a uniform helped staff to 'feel' professional. So, for example, the act of putting on scrubs may help staff to identify with the role and with a professional persona that they hope to portray to others. The wearing of a uniform was also linked to cleanliness and appearance, and in the minds of some participants how one looked and dressed extended beyond the boundaries of work. Many institutional policies refers to the legal context, which may apply to the wearing of appropriate dress from the perspective of health and safety and infection control, and may relate to issues of equality (in terms of age, disability, sex, sexual orientation, race, pregnancy and maternity, religion or belief and human rights). The Department of Health (DH) (2010a) has produced specific guidelines that provide detailed information on the legislation and the legal context of appropriate dress.

### Stop and think

How do you think that, as an ODP, dress code policies could apply to you, perhaps in clinical practice or, if you are a student, also at university?

In summary, taking into consideration the range of professional attributes and behaviours, a key feature is that of context itself. This includes the role and organization, for example, the NHS or independent healthcare sector, or the workplace such as the operating theatre, and the specific intervention (procedure). The HCPC study (2011: 12) reported that this variability was connected to:

well established, or even innate, personal qualities and values. This creates a dynamic tension for developing and assessing professionalism, as it is both an extremely personal, internalised belief, while being very much situated in the immediate environment.

### Professional values and beliefs

The question of professionalism with regard to behavioural aspects has been highlighted by the recent events that took place at the Mid Staffordshire NHS Foundation Trust, and the poor standard of care that often centred on the values and attitudes of some of the staff; although it is difficult to imagine how this could occur in the perioperative environment. The ODP should be aware that accepted attitudes, which by any normal standard would be considered unprofessional can lead to an organizational culture that the Francis inquiry (2010b: 152) found condoned the unacceptable behaviours of bullying, lack of candour (openness and honesty) and denial by refusing to accept that anything was wrong.

The lack of professionalism displayed by some staff also extended to poor communication and attitudes toward patients, their families and indeed other visitors. Contrast this with the findings of a study conducted by Wilkinson et al. (2009), who identified positive professional attributes. These centred typically around:

- adherence to ethical practice;
- effective interactions with patients and service users;
- effective interactions with staff;
- reliability, and commitment to improvement.

**Table 10.1** The 6 C's vision and values for good care

| | |
|---|---|
| Care | Care is our core business and that of our organizations, and the care we deliver helps the individual person and improves the health of the whole community. Caring defines us and our work. People receiving care expect it to be right for them, consistently, throughout every stage of their life |
| Compassion | Compassion is how care is given through relationships based on empathy, respect and dignity; it can also be described as intelligent kindness, and is central to how people perceive their care |
| Competence | Competence means all those in caring roles must have the ability to understand an individual's health and social needs and the expertise, clinical and technical knowledge to deliver effective care and treatments based on research and evidence |
| Communication | Communication is central to successful caring relationships and to effective team working. Listening is as important as what we say and do and essential for 'no decision about me without me'. Communication is the key to a good workplace with benefits for those in our care and staff alike |
| Courage | Courage enables us to do the right thing for the people we care for, to speak up when we have concerns and to have the personal strength and vision to innovate and to embrace new ways of working |
| Commitment | A commitment to our patients and populations is a cornerstone of what we do. We need to build on our commitment to improve the care and experience of our patients, to take action to make this vision and strategy a reality for all and meet the health, care and support challenges ahead |

*Source:* adapted from *Compassion in Practice Nursing, Midwifery and Care Staff: Our Vision and Strategy* on behalf of the DH/NHS Commissioning Board (2012)

Out of the failings of Mid Staffordshire has emerged a set of core values, the so-called 6 C's, which on their own are not new concepts, but together they are designed to reinforce vision and values for good care delivery (DH: 2012). The 6 C's affirm what can be considered to be personal qualities that each individual brings to their professionalism. Words like caring, compassion, empathy, respect and dignity are used to describe what is expected of the professional.

The perioperative environment can often feel very intense, the high degree of technical competence that may be required, and the level of pressure that staff experience can make it feel rather clinical, and therefore dispassionate.

**Stop and think**

How do you focus on care and compassion in the normal course of your day, and reflect on your own communication especially with patients?

## Professional judgement and decision-making

Other ways of looking at professional values and characteristics stem from the ODPs' own moral and ethical viewpoints, and therefore how ODPs arrive at patient-centred decision making. While the law influences value judgements, they also develop from social and cultural norms, for example, from our beliefs, religion and upbringing. ODPs might find that some of the clinical decisions that they are involved in, while legally and ethically acceptable, may not fit with their own moral viewpoint. Indeed, there may be times when ODPs are asked to do something or participate in a particular way of working that they are not comfortable with. As long as they reach an informed and reasonable decision based on the interests of the patient, and that they are able to justify this, it is likely that they would not be in breach of any regulatory standards.

### Moral and ethical dilemmas

Such conflicts, or dilemmas, should lead the ODP to consider how they undertake clinical decision making in the interests of the patient. In situations where such ambiguity exists, Griffith and Tengnah (2010) argue that it is essential that professional dilemmas are understood in order to make the right decisions to inform one's professional practice, particularly where these may well conflict with personal values. For example, an ODP might have a moral objection to certain surgical procedures (such as termination of pregnancy versus the sanctity of life). Equally, ODPs might not agree with a patient's decision to refuse further surgery; indeed, it might be the case that the ODP may think that further surgery would not be in the best interests of the patient.

In these circumstances such moral dilemmas can benefit from the application of ethical principles. While the focus is to explore how professionals arrive at effective clinical decision making as a key professional activity, it is worth briefly considering such an ethical approach, although the issue of ethics in ODP practice is discussed in more detail in Chapter 7. Beauchamp and Childress (1989) is perhaps the most accessible and indeed widely applicable model to explore whether a professional action is right or wrong. The stages, or principles, included in the model in the context of the ODP are as follows:

- Respect for autonomy – can be considered as the ability of the patient to decide for themselves on their treatment.
- Nonmaleficence – an ethical obligation placed upon the ODP not to harm the patient at any stage during the process of caring for the patient.
- Beneficence – challenges the ODP at all times to act in the best interests of the patient, so as to promote their wellbeing.
- Justice – requires the ODP to treat the patient fairly and impartially.

(adapted from Beauchamp and Childress, 1989)

For the ODP, such professional decision making should ensure that the patient has benefited from informed consent and that those caring for them are doing so according to the ODP's legal and professional duty. The HCPC's (2008) *Confidentiality – a Guidance for Registrants* has been produced to enable all registrants to reach informed and reasonable decisions.

Given the dynamic and changing context of perioperative practice, ODPs should strive to work within the limits of their competence. ODPs should stop and think how they can take account of feedback and peer review. Here appraisal mechanisms, mentorship and supervision can prove useful. ODPs have both a personal and professional obligation, and responsibility to recognize any deficits in their own skills and knowledge. This also extends to challenging incompetence and poor practice in others, as well as confronting any actions that risk bringing the profession into disrepute, and as the 6C's clearly state, have the courage and commitment to confront poor practice. The HCPC have made available as an e-resource, guidance to registrants on *Whistleblowing* (2013a) and *Raising and Escalating an Issue of Concern in the Workplace* (2013b).

### Stop and think

Consider if you have the courage and commitment to speak up to improve the patient's experience. How would you go about raising your concerns surrounding poor care?

### Clinical reasoning as a professional competence

The skill of the ODP in being able to relate and communicate effectively with patients can undoubtedly reduce patient anxiety, and this, in turn, can impact upon the psychological and physical response of the patient experiencing an anaesthetic, or surgical intervention. Atkins and Ersser (2008) argue that not only are effective clinical reasoning skills necessary for ethical care, but they also directly influence clinical effectiveness.

Different models of professional practice convey differences in the degree of importance placed upon the relationship between patient and professional. The perioperative environment raises specific challenges to the notion of patient involvement, or participation in their own care and treatment. As an alternative, Charles et al. (1999) advocates a shared decision-making approach. In which the role of the healthcare professional is to guide and support the patient to reach the right decision for them. By contrast 'informed choice' stresses the positive benefits and risks of any given treatment as the key responsibility of the healthcare professional, and in the perioperative environment this tends to be the responsibility of the medical team. If this was to change, the development of clinical reasoning may require the ODP to act as a conduit and resource for information. Furthermore, a key professional responsibility is to be able to help educate the patient to enable them to get involved in their treatment (Entwistle, 2000). In short, ODPs should recognize further their potential contribution to the long-term health promotion and wellbeing of the patient.

## Accountability, the role of the regulatory and codes of conduct

Having explored the concept of the professions and emerging context of professionalism in a healthcare context, there is a need to focus on the role of the regulator and the area of accountability. However, an overview of the legal framework of accountability may be helpful.

The principle of accountability in healthcare is there primarily to ensure public protection from acts or omissions that might cause harm, although, as previously argued, the term is wrongly applied and can lead to an issue of confusion in practice (Wordsworth, 2007: 192). ODPs can be called to account if their conduct, and indeed competence, falls below the legal standard. In such cases a range of legal sanctions are available that aim to deter the ODP from misconduct or unlawful actions. If a practitioner is called to account for their actions, such cases will be heard in public to ensure that patients can be assured that only high professional standards will be accepted (Griffith and Tengnah, 2010). It is important to stress that this principle also applies to ODPs, and as such public scrutiny provides an opportunity for the profession as a whole, to learn from cases of misconduct or incompetence. The HCPC publish on their website a list of hearings and outcomes from cases that are concerned with a practitioner's fitness to practise.

### Stop and think

Think about your accountability as an ODP, and for what reasons might your fitness to practise be called into question?

### An overview of accountability to civil and criminal law

Although the subject of further and detailed exploration in Chapter 6, it is worth remembering that legal accountability extends to criminal action in cases where society deems such breaches to be unacceptable; these include indictable acts such as murder and manslaughter. It is also worth stressing that as a result of statutory regulation ODP is a protected title. Using it when you are not entitled to do so is a prosecutable offence, so in cases where individuals continue to work as ODPs but lapse their registration, this can carry a fine of up to £5,000 and lead to a criminal conviction and disclosure to employers and the HCPC (PSA, 2013). ODPs are also legally accountable to the civil courts and the laws of tort as actions between individuals, rather than with society as a whole. The area of practitioner negligence is particularly apposite here, as is the issue of consent, and confidentiality as a form of trespass. It is also important to note that negligence has been judged by the courts to be grossly negligent such that it is dealt with as a criminal matter (Montgomery, 2003). The case of *R v. Adomako* [1994], which will have a particular resonance with some ODPs, was settled by the House of Lords and involved an anaesthetist who, over a period of time, failed to notice that an endotracheal (ET) had become detached, resulting in the patient suffering a cardiac arrest. The Court of Appeal provided some clarity in defining the criteria, which should be applied to all health professions in such cases. This includes an obvious indifference on behalf of the health professional to any risks to the patient, and having known the obvious risks, the healthcare professional chooses to carry on without regard for the patient's safety.

Montgomery (2003: 188) describes how in cases of criminal negligence, 'attempts to avoid a known risk where grossly negligent that the jury believed that they deserved to be punished'. The bottom line is that healthcare professionals, ODPs included, are accountable to the criminal courts, and can be punished accordingly should a jury decide that such a sanction is necessary and deserved.

The third sphere of professional accountability is that of the ODP to their employer. All employees (ODPs included) are 'obliged to follow the lawful and reasonable instructions of their employers' (Montgomery, 2003: 19). However, it is the area of protocol or procedural compliance that is particularly important. Deviation from agreed protocols may indicate that there is a case of negligence to answer. In such cases, employees would also invariably find themselves subject to disciplinary action, culminating in possible dismissal. In the case of agency ODPs who are technically temporary staff employed through a third party, they are accountable to the agency as their employer, but under the conditions of their employment they must still comply with Trust policies and procedures. Matters of concern and issues of a disciplinary nature would be dealt with by the agency itself. Lastly, but of particular significance, ODPs could find that breaches in adherence to procedures could also lead to accusation of professional misconduct, linked with regulation, registration and standards.

### Stop and think

Think about how the failure to adhere to hospital policies and procedures could lead to employer sanctions, and or, legal action. Which policies do you feel are particularly relevant to you as an ODP?

### The HCPC and the ODP

ODPs are accountable to a 'higher authority' via the provisions of *The Health and Social Work Order 2001*, which itself was made under section 60 of the *Health Act 1999*. Although the former brought into being the HCPC, the inclusion of ODPs resulted from additional legislation in the form of *The Health Professions (Operating Department Practitioners and Miscellaneous Amendments)*.

The HCPC is an independent and multi-professional regulator (separate from the Government) and its purpose is to protect the public. It does this by primarily keeping a register of individuals, called 'registrants', from 16 separate professions. In order to remain registered, a registrant is expected to meet a number of standards used to determine an individual's fitness to practise. If the HCPC receive concerns over a registrant's fitness to practise, a preliminary investigation is undertaken to assess whether 'there is a case to answer'. If the answer is yes this will be referred to a hearing, which will take place in one of the following committees:

- conduct and competence committee (for cases about misconduct, lack of competence convictions or cautions, decisions by other regulators and barring decisions);
- a panel of the health committee (for cases where the health of the professional may be affecting their ability to practise).

In cases where there is evidence that a registrant's fitness to practise is impaired, The Health Professions Order (2001) 29 (c) makes provisions that enable either committee to:

(a) make an order directing the Registrar to strike the person concerned off the register (a "striking-off order").
(b) make an order directing the Registrar to suspend the registration of the person concerned for a specified period which shall not exceed one year (a "suspension order").
(c) make an order imposing conditions with which the person concerned must comply for a specified period which shall not exceed three years (a "conditions of practice order"); or
(d) caution the person concerned and make an order directing the Registrar to annotate the register accordingly for a specified period which shall be not less than one year and not more than five years (a "caution order").

There are seven sets of standards, although not all apply to the registrant or the ODP profession. *Standards of Education and Training (SETs)* set out the requirements for training that apply to the education provider. Whereas, the *Standards for Prescribing* are linked to specific legislation that enables some professions to act as prescribers, at present the legal framework does not allow for ODPs to be either 'supplementary' or 'independent prescribers'. Two further standards are concerned with *character* and *health* but are related to the *Standards of Conduct, Performance and Ethics.*

- *Character* – joining the register is subject to a character check to ensure that the applicant can practise 'safely and effectively'. At the point of joining the register, an applicant must inform the HCPC about any criminal convictions or cautions. Once registered 'registrants' have a responsibility to inform the HCPC if they are subsequently convicted or cautioned (HCPC: 2013c).
- *Health – Standard 12 of the Standards of Conduct, Performance, and Ethics* states that, 'You must limit your work or stop practising if your performance or judgement is affected by your health.' This standard is also used to make judgements about disability or long-term health conditions. This need not be a barrier to a career in the health professions regulated by the HCPC, as long as the applicant has the necessary insight to manage and understand their condition without impairing their ability to practise safely (HCPC, 2013d).

  The *Standards of Conduct, Performance and Ethics* are generic standards of behaviour, which express public and professional expectations of each of the HCPC's registrants. These define the regulatory basis on which the ODPs values, behaviour and character are based. They codify many of the attributes that were previously identified in the HCPC (2011) study on professionalism. They also guide the ODP to enable them to arrive at the right decisions in their conduct and care of the patient. Standard 13 places a regulatory responsibility on the ODP registrant such that: 'You must behave with honesty and integrity and make sure that your behaviour does not damage the public's confidence in you or your profession' (HCPC: 2012a).

These standards apply to those wishing to enter the register, therefore student ODPs should stop and think how non-compliance can reasonably affect their ability to register and work as an ODP. The HCPC (2012b) has also produced *Guidance on Conduct and Ethics for Students.* Further specific information for ODP students is available from CODP (2013), in the form of *Student Professional Obligations. Both* mirror the *Standards of Conduct, Performance and Ethics.*

The *Standards of Proficiency (SoPs) for Operating Department Practice* are threshold standards to be achieved at the point of registration. Students who have completed a recognized training programme should be aware that they are not registered automatically, but are eligible to apply for entry onto the register (subject to meeting the conditions of good health and character). Once registered ODPs must be able to demonstrate, at the point of renewal (or re-enter to the register) that they continue to meet the SoPs. The SoPs contain generic standards as key obligations that apply to all HCPC registrants; as well as profession specific standards that together define the knowledge, specific skills, and competences needed to continue to practise safely and effectively (HCPC, 2014). This can also be regarded as the ODPs' *Scope of Practice*, which may well be different for each ODP according to their role, experience and institution that they work in.

The HCPC's (2012c) *Your Guide to our Standards for Continuing Professional Development (CPD)* in effect links the ability of the ODP to be able to meet the SoPs. These standards provide a mechanism by which the registrant can maintain, update and record their professional development throughout their careers. Readers should refer to Chapter 11 for a more detailed and contextual exploration of the CPD in relation to ODPs.

### Stop and think

What kinds of activity are you involved in that could count as CPD. Thinking about the SoPs, are there any current areas of your practice that need particularly updating?

## The Scope of Practice for ODPs

Given the professional context of the perioperative environment, including changes to medical staffing and training of junior doctors, technology and patient demographics, it is reasonable to assume that the role of the ODP will continue to develop over time. The extent of this development, including the development of roles outside of the operating theatre, covers the following roles:

- surgical care practitioner;
- surgical pre-assessment practitioner;
- physician's assistant;
- resuscitation officer;
- transplant co-ordinator;
- specialist ophthalmic anaesthetic practitioner.

The development of the scope of practice of the profession and context of these developments has led the CODP (2010: 5) to consider how the ODP can remain clinically effective:

As the healthcare environment continues to change, practitioners are required to maintain and develop their competence, to develop their knowledge base as knowledge changes and expand, and to adapt their skills to new circumstances in which they find themselves. In preparation for their role, the pre-registration education of ODPs, as for other healthcare professions, must take account of the challenging environment of care; it must continue to prepare practitioners who are fit for purpose, fit for practice and fit for award.

To this end the CODP (2011) have embarked on a radical overhaul of curriculum (which defines the 'body of knowledge' and articulates with the HCPC's SoPs). As the CODP acknowledge, there is little doubt that changes in the scope of practice for the profession as a whole are reflected in the attempts of the higher education institutes (HEIs) to ensure that their programmes are regularly subject to review and re-approval in order to remain current and contemporary. Nevertheless, in moving to a degree-level curriculum, CODP (2010: 6) make the case that: 'It is no longer possible, however, to expect such "ad-hoc" adaptations to continue to be effective; the time has arrived for a major revision of the ODP curriculum.'

Many ODPs specialize in a particular area (anaesthetics, surgery, post-anaesthetic care), and sub-specialism (such as paediatrics, neurosurgery, cardio-thoracic, vascular). Indeed, roles that focus on management, education and research are far more common than once was, meaning that the ODP may not be able to meet all of the SoPs. This should not pose a problem given that the ODP exercises their professional judgement and does not practise in activities that they are not competent or proficient in. The HCPC recognizes that ODPs are autonomous professionals, and as such they expect them to arrive at informed and reasonable decisions to ensure that standards continue to be met. At times this might be achieved in different ways and ODPs should know when to seek advice where appropriate. The CODP (2009: 7) has produced guidance to enable ODPs to understand their scope of practice, and if necessary extend it. Their specific advice encourages the ODP to undertake the following self-assessment in order to comply with legal, ethical and regulatory mechanisms of accountability:

- Do I consider that I am participating in a reasonable and justifiable course of treatment or intervention?
- Am I aware of, and have considered, any evidenced-based practice?
- In order to participate competently in the care of the patient, do I have the necessary knowledge, skills and experience?
- Am I able to demonstrate professional development and fitness for practise through maintaining my CPD?

Importantly, from April 2014, ODPs are required, as a condition of remaining on the HCPC register, to declare that they have 'appropriate' professional indemnity in place. This is normally the case for those working in the NHS; however, ODPs participating in an area of extended scope of practice should check that this remains the case. ODPs working in the independent sector, or through an agency, should put in place their own arrangements.

## Advanced practice and the ODP

Given the context of the profession, and the changes that are taking place in healthcare, it is not surprising that the role of the ODP is changing. However, the advancement of practice raises a number of important legal and professional matters. These developments are likely to mean that issues such as the responsibility for delegation and supervision come to the fore as individuals adapt their own scope of practice (either as specialists or managers), and as the profession adopts practices and responsibilities that were once the preserve mainly of the medical profession. Changes in the working practices and employment contracts of junior doctors in moving away from the apprentice-ship model have radically altered the way that hospitals are staffed (McGee, 2009a). This is particularly evident in the operating theatre; however, the full impact of this I suspect has not been felt.

### Delegation and supervision

Managerial or leadership activities in the operating theatre (up to now the most obvious route for advanced practice in ODP) can be complex and challenging. Although responsibility remains with those in charge, failure to carry this out effectively can have legal consequences if tasks are delegated to staff who do not have the experience or training to undertake them safely (Dimond, 2002).

It is worth pointing out that there is no provision for team liability, and the courts have rejected the 'captain of the ship' doctrine where one individual takes sole responsibility for the 'acts or omissions of others'. As Dimond (2002) argues, each professional is accountable for their actions and is central to the determination of professional negligence. The legal standard for this, and for the HCPC, would be to apply the principles set out according to the Bolam test, or what is expected of the 'ordinary skilled person' (see Chapter 6). However, in practice, the law requires a higher standard from a healthcare profession than members of the general public, so the ODP would be judged according to the minimum level of competence expected of the ODP. However, the courts have established that someone who is junior, or not as experienced, should provide the same standard of care as those who normally carry out the role. In effect there is no defence for inexperience as seen in *Nettleship* v. *Weston* (1971).

### Surgical care practitioners and physicians assistants

The principles of delegation and supervision are also applicable where an activity is delegated to a different profession, say an ODP working as a physician's assistant. In that case they would be judged according to the minimum level of competence of the doctor who normally carries out that function (see *Wilsher* v. *Essex Area Health Authority*). Wall (2004), in effect, points out that the standard should reflect the post and not the post-holder. Samanta and Samanta (2011) raise such concerns over the delegated role of the surgical care practitioner working under the direction and supervision of a surgeon (see also Freudmann and Aning, 2006). However, in situations where supervision is provided, the practitioner may discharge their duty of care if they acknowledge that they lack the necessary expertise, and therefore seek advice from those with more experience. This is problematic however, as knowing when to refer naturally requires experience, and indeed some considerable expertise. The role of the physician's assistant includes complex roles and decision making around diagnosis, treatment and autonomous intervention (DH, 2006). However, McGee (2009b: 9) points out that in contrast to the advanced nurse practitioner, the doctor continues to be responsible for, and supervises the physician's assistant according to a medical model.

### Stop and think

Think about your own scope of practice and what you need to do in order to maintain, or develop it?

## Prescribing and advanced practice

The drafting of *The Misuse of Drugs and the Misuse of Drugs (Safe Custody) (Amendment) Regulations 2007* has clarified that ODPs are authorized to possess and supply Schedules 2 to 5 controlled drugs in accordance with the prescriber (see Chapter 6). However, at present ODPs are not able to act as supplementary or independent prescribers and they are not one of the professions who are entitled to participate in patient group directions (PGDs). It is likely that in the near future CODP may wish to lobby for changes to these rules, as there is growing anecdotal evidence that by not enabling ODPs to participate in PGDs, this has detrimental consequences to patient-centred care and patient outcomes, both in the form of delays to treatment and the quality of care, as well as the responsiveness, efficacy and efficiency of treatment.

The skill set of the ODP should be highly transferable to future advanced roles and responsibilities; however, this is potentially compromised by not being able to take part in PGDs or prescribing. While Shortland and Hardware (2009) point out, that the ability to prescribe does not necessarily constitute advanced practice, a growing number of ODPs' scope of practice does include advanced clinical skills such as patient assessment, history taking, treatment planning, and autonomous diagnosis and intervention. Therefore, the omission of ODPs from functions that involve full access to medicines administration, can not only affect the patient, but also disadvantages some individual ODPs who cannot practice in advanced roles despite having the skills and knowledge to do so. Furthermore, these limitations restrict the opportunities for intra-professional working, and highlight the disparities between different professions such as ODPs and theatre nurses who essentially are carrying out the same role.

## Conclusion

The view as to whether the ODP can now be classed as a profession, given the contemporary discourse surrounding the emphasis on 'professionalism', is perhaps a moot point. Given the characteristics that have surfaced in these new debates, 'grand theories' that have always defied agreement and consensus are being replaced by identifiable characteristics that are not necessarily based on hierarchy or status. Therefore, the question as to whether regulation has changed the way that ODPs practise is down to individual qualities and the perception of themselves as professionals.

Apart from the growing importance of values and behaviours as a key professional concern in their own right, these are clearly linked to the ODPs' accountability from a legal and regulatory perspective. Adherence to standards and codes of conduct is part of the contract, over and above the law, that the profession makes with the public to ensure that they remain confident that they will be treated and cared for in a competent and compassionate way. Moreover, there are consequences for ODPs, and students alike, where such standards fall short of what is expected.

In the context of contemporary healthcare, it is likely that the ODPs' scope of practice is potentially open to development, either individually, or to the profession in its entirety. Knowing when to develop, or advance one's role is itself a professional characteristic, and having highlighted examples of this, challenging accepted practice and ways of working requires the ODP to be cognizant of their own accountability. That said, hurdles still remain and these should be challenged where appropriate. Therefore, it is hoped that this chapter will stimulate such debates and act as a catalyst for further investigation and research from other ODPs in order to inform and advance their own patient-centred practice and indeed the profession as a whole.

### Key points

- Professionalism should be viewed as a set of characteristics and qualities that transcend professional status and hierarchy.
- Demonstrating the right values and behaviours should be central to the ODPs professional practice.
- Accountability is an important consequence of professionalism that links to professional and legal standards of conduct and competence.
- The scope of practice relates to both professional and individual practitioners roles, both of which should be expected to change and develop.
- Advanced practice has the potential to improve the care of the patient but for the ODP some barriers still remain.

### List of cases

Nettleship v. Weston [1971] QB 691 (CA)
R v. Adomako [1994] 1 AC 171 (HL)
Wilsher v. Essex Area Health Authority [1988] AC 1074 (HL)

**References and further reading**

Association of Operating Department Practitioners (AODP) (2001) *DipHE in Operating Department Practice, Curriculum Document.* Lewes: AODP.

Atkins, S. and Ersser, J.S. (2008) 'Clinical reasoning and patient-centred care', in Higgs, J., Jones, M.A., Loftus, S. and Christensen, N. (eds) *Clinical Reasoning in the Health Professions* (3rd edn). London: Elsevier, Butterworth, Heinmann.

Beauchamp. T. and Childress, J. (1989) *Principle of Biomedical Ethics.* Oxford: Oxford University Press.

Bourdieu, P. (1984) *Distinction: A Social Critique of the Judgement of Taste,* translated by Nice, R. London: Routledge and Kegan Paul.

Bourdieu, P. (2006) 'The forms of capital', in Lauder, H., Brown, P., Dillaborough, J.A. and Halsey, A.H. (eds) *Education, Globalisation and Social Change.* Oxford: Oxford University Press.

Charles, C., Gafni, A. and Whelan, T. (1999) 'Decision-making in the physician-patient encounter: revisiting the shared treatment decision-making model', *Social Sciences and Medicine,* 49: 651–61.

College of Operating Department Practitioners (CODP) (2009) *Scope of Practice.* London: CODP.

College of Operating Department Practitioners (CODP) (2010) *Discussion Paper – Framing the Future Role and Function of Operating Department Practitioners.* London: CODP.

College of Operating Department Practitioners (CODP) (2011) *Bachelor of Science (Hons) in Operating Department Practice – England, Northern Ireland and Wales,* Curriculum Document, London: CODP.

College of Operating Department Practitioners (CODP) (2013) *Students Standards of Professional Behaviour.* London: CODP.

Cruess, R.L. and Cruess, S.R. (2006) 'Teaching professionalism: general principles', *Medical Teacher,* 28: 205–08.

Curry, G. and Suhomlinova, O. (2006) 'The impact of institutional forces upon knowledge sharing in the UK NHS: the triumph of professional power and the inconsistency of policy', *Public Administration,* 84 (1): 1–30.

Department of Health (DH) (2006) *The Competence and Curriculum Framework for the Physicians Assistant.* London: DH.

Department of Health (DH) (2010a) *Uniforms and Workwear: Guidance on Uniform and Workwear Policies for NHS Employers.* Available online at http://webarchive.nationalarchives.gov. uk/20130107105354/http://www.dh.gov.uk/prod_consum_dh/groups/dh_digitalassets/@dh/ @en/@ps/documents/digitalasset/dh_114754.pdf (accessed 28 September 2013).

Department of Health (DH) (2010b) *The Mid Staffordshire NHS Foundation Trust Inquiry.* London: DH>

Department of Health (DH)/NHS Commissioning Board (2012) *Compassion in Practice Nursing, Midwifery and Care Staff: Our Vision and Strategy.* Available online at http://www.england.nhs.uk/ wp-content/uploads/2012/12/compassion-in-practice.pdf (accessed 23 Septemder 2013).

Dimond, B. (2002) *Legal Aspects of Radiography and Radiology.* Oxford: Blackwell Science Ltd.

Elston, A.M. (1991) 'The politics of professional power: medicine in a changing health service', in Gabe, J., Calnan, M. and Bury, M. (eds) *The Sociology of the Health Service.* London: Routledge.

Entwistle, V.A. (2000) 'Supporting and resourcing treatment decision-making; some policy considera-tion', *Health Expectations,* 3: 77–85.

Foucault, M. (1977) *Discipline and Punishment: The Birth of the Prison.* London: Penguin Press.

Freudmann, M. and Aning, J. (2006) 'Surgical care practitioners are having a detrimental effect on surgical training', *British Medical Journal (BMJ).* Available online at http://careers.bmj.com/ careers/advice/bmj.333.7567.s97.xml (accessed 7 September 2012).

Friedson, E. (1994) *Professions Reborn: Theory, Prophecy and Policy*. Cambridge: Polity Press.

Griffith, R. and Tengnah, C. (2010) *Law and Professional Issues in Nursing* (2nd edn). Exeter: Learning Matters.

Health Act (1999) London: HMSO. Available online at http://www.legislation.gov.uk/ukpga/1999/8/contents (accessed 7 September 2013).

Health and Care Professions Council (HCPC) (2008) *Confidentiality – a Guidance for Registrants*. London: HCPC.

Health and Care Professions Council (HCPC) (2010) *Guidance on Conduct and Ethics for Students*. Available online at http://www.hpc-uk.org/assets/documents/10002C16Guidanceonconductandethicsforstudents.pdf (accessed 7 September 2013).

Health and Care Professions Council (HCPC) (2011) *Professionalism in the Health Professions, Research Report*. London: HCPC.

Health and Care Professions Council (HCPC) (2012a) *Standards of Conduct, Performance and Ethics*. London: HCPC.

Health and Care Professions Council (HCPC) (2012b) *Guidance on Conduct and Ethics for Students*, London: HCPC.

Health and Care Professions Council (HCPC) (2012c) *Your Guide to our Standards of Continuing Professional Development*. HCPC: London.

Health and Care Professions Council (HCPC) (2012d) *Standards of Education and Training*. London: HCPC.

Health and Care Professions Council (HCPC) (2013a) *Whistleblowing*. Available online at http://www.hpc-uk.org/registrants/raisingconcerns/whistleblowing/ (accessed 7 September 2013).

Health and Care Professions Council (HCPC) (2013b) *Raising and Escalating Concerns in the Workplace*. Available online at http://www.hpc-uk.org/registrants/raisingconcerns/ (accessed 7 September 2013).

Health and Care Professions Council (HCPC) (2013c) *Character*. Available online at http://www.hpc-uk.org/aboutregistration/standards/character/ (accessed 7 September 2013).

Health and Care Professions Council (HCPC) (2013d) *Health*. Available online at http://www.hpc-uk.org/aboutregistration/standards/health/ (accessed 7 September 2013).

Health and Care Professions Council (HCPC) (2014) *Standards of Proficiency – Operating Department Practitioners*. London: HCPC.

Macdonald, M.K. (1995) *The Sociology of the Professions*. London: Sage Publications.

McGee, P. (2009a) 'The development of advanced nursing practice in the United Kingdom', in McGee, P. (ed.) *Advanced Practice in Nursing and the Allied Health Profession* (3rd edn). Chichester: Wiley-Blackwell.

McGee, P. (2009b) 'The future of advanced practice', in McGee, P. (ed.) *Advanced Practice in Nursing and the Allied Health Profession* (3rd edn). Chichester: Wiley-Blackwell.

Montgomery, J. (2003) *Health Care Law* (2nd edn.) Oxford: Oxford University Press.

National Health Service Executive (NHS Executive) (2000) *The Employment of Operating Department Practitioners* (ODPs), Guidance in the NHS Letter dated 20 March 2000. London: NHS Executive.

Professional Standards Authority (PSA) (2013) *Lapses in Professional Registration: Impact, Issues, and Ideas for Improvement*. London: PSA for Health and Social Care.

Reay, D., David, E.M. and Ball, S. (2005) *Degrees of Choice: Social Class, Race and Gender in Higher Education*. Stoke-on-Trent: Trentham Books.

Samanta, J. and Samanta, A. (2011) *Medical Law*. Basingstoke: Palgrave Macmillan.

Shortland, S. and Hardware, K. (2009) 'Prescribing and advanced practice', in McGee, P. (ed.) *Advanced Practice in Nursing and the Allied Health Profession* (3rd edn). Chichester: Wiley-Blackwell.

Stern, D.T (2006) (ed.) *Measuring Medical Professionalism*. Oxford: Oxford University Press.

The Health Professions (Operating Department Practitioners and Miscellaneous Amendments) Order 2004. Available online at http://www.legislation.gov.uk/uksi/2004/2033/contents/made (accessed 31 August 2013).

The Health Professions Order 2001. Available online at http://www.legislation.gov.uk/uksi/2002/254/article/29/made (accessed 7 September 2013).

The Mid Staffordshire NHS Foundation Trust Inquiry (2010) *Independent Inquiry into Care Provided by Mid Staffordshire NHS Foundation Trust January 2005–March 2009*, Volume I, Chaired by Robert Francis QC. London: HMSO.

The Misuse of Drugs and the Misuse of Drugs (Safe Custody) (Amendment) Regulations 2007. Available online at http://www.legislation.gov.uk/uksi/2007/2154/contents/made (accessed 8 September 2013).

Timmons, S. (2011) 'Professionalization and its discontents', *Health: An Interdisciplinary, Journal for the Study of Health, Illness and Medicine*, 15 (4): 337–52.

Timmons, S. and Tanner, J. (2004) 'A disputed occupational boundary: operating theatre nurses and Operating Department Practitioners', *Sociology of Health & Illness*, 26 (5): 645–66.

Wall, I. (2004) 'Clinical negligence', in Payne-James, J., Dean, P. and Wall, I. (eds) *Medicolegal Essentials in Healthcare* (2nd edn). London: GMM.

Weber, M. (1978) *Economy and Society*. London: The University of California Press.

Wilkinson, T., Wade, W.B. and Knock, L.D. (2009) 'A blueprint to assess professionalism: results of a systematic review', *Academic Medicine*, 84: 551– 58.

Witz, A. (1992) *Professions and Patriarchy*. London: Routledge.

Wordsworth, S. (2007) 'Accountability in peri-operative practice', in Smith, B., Rawling, P., Wicker, P. and Jones, S. (eds) *Core Topics in Operating Department Practice: Anaesthesia and Critical Care*. Cambridge: Cambridge University Press.

Wordsworth, S. (2011) Student choice in the allied health professions, paper presented at the Centre for Health and Social Care Annual Research Conference, Birmingham City University.

# 11 Lifelong learning and continuous professional development for the Operating Department Practitioner

## Susan Parker

**Key topics**

- Professionalization and continuous professional development (CPD)

- Why CPD?

- Defining lifelong learning and CPD

- Exploring CPD and the benefits of this

- Which forms of learning constitute CPD?

- Planning and managing your CPD

- What if I am selected by the Health Care and Professions Council (HCPC) to submit my CPD profile?

## Introduction

The profession of Operating Department Practitioners (ODPs) has undergone a series of rapid and successive changes: changes that have brought CPD to the forefront of our professional practice. Prior to its introduction as a prerequisite of professional regulation, many ODPs may not have been actively engaged in learning beyond the requirements of their immediate roles and practice contexts. This chapter explores the concepts and practices of CPD through defining what CPD actually is; examining the nature of its relationship to professional practice and its importance as a measure of our competence set against an increasingly complex and dynamically changing healthcare environment.

## Why is this relevant?

The healthcare environment is constantly changing and this is no more apparent than within the perioperative environment where medical care and surgical treatment is advancing rapidly with the introduction of new innovations, procedures and equipment to treat and manage patients. In order to retain currency and credibility against the changing nature of healthcare practices, our own profession of ODPs led by the College of Operating Department Practitioners (CODP) have undergone a series of changes. The introduction of the Diploma of Higher Education (DipHE) in Operating Department Practice in 2001 saw a more academic approach to education for the profession, as higher education institutes (HEIs) became the sole providers of the pre-registration qualification.

These changes to the delivery of pre-registration education for ODPs were met with some criticism and discontent as there was a perceived erosion of the deep-seated relationship with the practical dimensions of the ODP role as some thought the DipHE programme was creating a theory/practice divide, an observable fact that also occurred within nursing with the introduction of Project 2000 (Maben et al., 2006).

Although there was initial disquiet, there has been a subsequent and significant shift in culture and attitude towards the changes as the advantages and benefits became more and more apparent; and the most observable benefit may be considered the creation of increased opportunities for ODPs. The opportunities for widening the scope of practice both within and outside of the usual perioperative environments has meant that ODPs are no longer confined to their anaesthetic rooms as once was the tradition and can be increasingly found occupying some diverse roles both within and outside of the healthcare sector. This has been in part due to the unique and valuable range of clinical skills, specialist knowledge, adaptability and experiences. This has meant that the opportunities for ODPs to develop and diversify are continually increasing.

The changes to the pre-registration education of ODPs occurred around the time of the attainment of professional regulation by the HCPC in 2004. One of the most significant changes, which came as part of this statutory regulation by the HCPC, was the introduction of mandatory CPD for all registrants from July 2006. The rationale for its introduction was founded on the basis that it formed an important dimension of professional self-regulation, and one that linked with the primary function in protecting the health and wellbeing of the public (HCPC, 2004). In accordance with the HCPC *Standards of Conduct, Performance and Ethics*, it is our responsibility as a registrant to ensure that our knowledge, skills and performance within our own areas of practice are of a high quality and up to date (HCPC, 2012a). The importance of engaging in career-long, self-directed learning as a mechanism of maintaining fitness to practise is clearly stated in our *Standards of Proficiency* (HCPC, 2014).

## Professionalization and CPD

We often hear the phrase 'trust me, I'm a professional' but what does it actually mean to be a professional and in particular a healthcare professional? What defines us as ODPs? Or sets us apart from other occupational groups?

Within the literature, health and social care professions are often referred to as 'caring professions', which Ellis defines as 'intending to identify a group of professions that have characteristics in common and are distinguishable from others' (Ellis, 1998: 43). In reviewing the definitions of a profession from across the literature a number of characteristics are distinguishable and ones that ODPs reflect:

- a distinct body of knowledge;
- monitoring and validation of education and training programmes;
- register of members and self-regulation through the relevant professional body;
- codes of conduct and ethics, and participation in a subculture sustained by the professional associations;
- engagement in CPD to demonstrate competence and fitness to practise.

A number of these characteristics have been explored in Chapter 10; however, the final defining characteristic of being a professional is the requirement to engage in CPD. This, according to extensive and ongoing research undertaken by Friedman et al. (2008: 7) into learning within a professional context, 'doing CPD is part of what defines (us) as professionals'. And thus the nature and relationship of CPD extends to become an intrinsic part of our identity and part of our everyday working practices. It is also a process that not only enables us to re-register with the HCPC, but is a measure of our ongoing competence and fitness to practise. Failure to submit evidence of our learning activities on request, or demonstrate a sufficient range of CPD, can also result in suspension or removal from the register. The relevance and importance of engaging in regular CPD therefore cannot be overemphasized.

## Why CPD?

New knowledge, new procedures, new processes and new environments will enforce new thinking, new actions and new ideas. A professional person who does not understand and implement the need for continuous improvement in a lifelong learning world is not just standing still; they are falling behind (Longworth, 2003: 130).

It has long been recognized that our initial training and qualification is insufficient to meet the needs and expectations of a changing society (Roscoe, 2002). The knowledge and skills with which each ODP begins their career has a short 'shelf life', with Watkins (1999) estimating that the lifespan of the knowledge obtained through a vocational qualification is approximately four years. Many ODPs, especially those who trained under the older (pre-diploma) awards, may not have formalized their CPD or recorded it appropriately as their CPD activities may have been centred on the requirements of their immediate roles/responsibilities/needs. However, roles have expanded and responsibilities increased, which has led to an increasing expectation for ODPs to take responsibility for managing both their career pathways as well as planning their own learning needs to ensure they retain currency within their roles. Participation in CPD has become an integral part of ODPs' practice that serves to fulfil a number of requirements.

## Defining lifelong learning and CPD

Lifelong learning and CPD are both well-established principles that drive the ongoing education, training and development of many healthcare professions (Department of Health (DH), 2004) including ODPs. The two terms are often used interchangeably and do share some common characteristics in serving to encompass a full range of learning activities, contributing to personal development as well as benefiting wider social dimensions. It is however important to consider the distinction between these principles for the ODP to meet both their professional and employment requirements.

Lifelong learning is a fairly broad term that is used by governments and other organizations to meet the challenges of globalization amid the emergence of a knowledge-based economy. From the National Health Service (NHS) perspective, therefore, lifelong learning is considered crucial in enabling the delivery of the government's vision of a world-class healthcare service (DH, 2012). The NHS displays commitment to lifelong learning principles through its numerous policies that reiterate the valuable contribution learning, in all its forms, makes to practitioners' everyday working practices particularly in enhancing patient care and achieving local and national strategic objectives. The importance of training, education and development is perhaps more evident since the NHS has been placed under increased scrutiny following the Francis Report (2013). Regular audits of hospitals on behalf of the Care Quality Commission (CQC) monitor patient service, quality and experiences, including operating theatres, with education and training forming a major component of these audits. The NHS Constitution (DH, 2010) highlights the commitment to providing staff with personal development opportunities in order to undertake their roles and it has been recognized that there is a link between healthcare education and the delivery of safe patient care (NPSA, 2004). The NHS has also emphasized the importance of teaching non-technical skills such as communication and teamworking to directly address patient safety issues and this is evident in the perioperative environment through the introduction of the WHO Surgical Safety Checklist (National Patient Safety Agency (NPSA), 2009) and Human Factors Training (www.patientsafetyfirst.nhs.uk) which are both high-profile initiatives with specific focus on operating department practice.

CPD is a process by which ODPs regularly demonstrate that they are meeting professional responsibilities, and maintaining competence and fitness to practise. It provides a framework that enables ODPs to meet the growing demand for quality, competence and accountability and ensures that patients receive the best possible care. In addition, it serves to help ODPs to respond to ongoing changes both within the individual's own practice areas as well as the wider challenges of healthcare provision.

Current pre-registration programmes of study integrate the concept of professional issues including the importance of CPD for use beyond registration. Biggs and Tang (2011), in their exploration of healthcare-related programmes, recognize the importance of lifelong learning principles and emphasize the relationship between the clinical and academic environments stating that 'lifelong learning is a broad concept that interfaces between institution and workplace from pre-university to continuing professional development after graduation' (Biggs and Tang, 2011: 160).

## Stop and think

Thinking about your current role:

What organizational/departmental/procedural changes (if any) have you experienced over the past year?

How have they affected you and how have you adapted to these changes?

Were there any training or support mechanisms in place to help you meet these changes?

## Focusing on CPD?

Although CPD shares commonalities with lifelong learning, and occupies a unique position on the lifelong learning continuum, it possesses a number of distinct features. Whereas lifelong learning is portrayed as being inclusive of all learning from 'cradle to grave', CPD is a process of structured, specific learning and development, determined and undertaken by an individual during the 'practitioner's working life' (Megginson and Whittaker, 2007: 5) and involves aspects of reflection, action and importantly application to practice. It has furthermore become synonymous with professionalism and development of professional identity, with learning governed by professional standards.

The term 'continuous professional development' (CPD) is attributed to Richard Gardner who was responsible for professional development within the building professions at York University during the 1970s. His intention was the introduction of a framework of professional development that sought to re-establish the links between education and practice, which he saw as lacking in post-qualified practising professionals (Gardner, 1978). Gardner furthermore recognized the multidimensional nature of knowledge advocated by Schön (1983) that serves to encompass technical, process, professional and tacit knowledge, as well as reiterating the importance of informal, work-based and incidental learning that we engage in through our everyday practices. CPD was, in his view, also a formal and more public way of organizing what professionals did informally as part of their working lives. Recognizing the value of CPD led to the adoption and introduction of CPD policies across a number of professional bodies during the late 1990s.

A wealth of definitions of CPD can be found in the literature from Early and Bubb's elegantly simple and straightforward description as a process that 'encompasses all formal and informal learning that enables individuals to improve their practice' (Earley and Bubb, 2007: 3) to more in-depth and profession-specific ones. The professional regulator for ODPs, the HCPC, defines CPD as:

a range of learning activities through which professionals maintain and develop throughout their career to ensure that they retain their capacity to practise safely, effectively and legally within their evolving scope of practice.

(Allied Health Professions Project, 2002, cited in HCPC 2012b: 1)

Our own profession-generic definition predominantly focuses on the individual practitioner, their responsibilities and obligations to practise within their defined roles under *The Standards of Conduct, Performance and Ethics* (HCPC, 2012a). While other professions are required to undertake a specific number of hours or gather a designated number points as evidence of their CPD activities, the HCPC decided to opt for a less prescriptive approach. It was their view that due to the differing nature of the individual registrants and their diverse roles, each practitioner would be able to dedicate different amounts of time to learning (HCPC, 2004). There was also the possibility that learning could become a points-gathering exercise which, in turn, would negate any meaning or value attached to the learning.

Although broadness and flexibility exists regarding the 'range of learning activities' deemed relevant by the HCPC, it further acknowledges the variation of ODPs' individual roles, responsibilities and learning needs while still adhering to the need to meet professional standards. The definition further alludes to wider contexts of practice and the increasing relationships within and outside of the organization as our roles and scope of practice may move beyond our current defined boundaries.

The terms *future* and *evolving scope of practice* signpost not only individuals' potential achievements but acknowledges and sanctions the changing healthcare workforce and practices. The ODP as a knowledgeable worker is required to adjust to new and evolving situations as government targets and initiatives challenge our current roles and responsibilities. And as changes are becoming more frequent, the importance of measurable CPD becomes more imperative.

Although we 'know' or have our own idea what CPD constitutes, and recognize it as an accepted and intrinsic component of our professional identity and practice, research concludes that CPD is not a straightforward concept. Its ambiguous nature results from the 'definitional variety between professional associations' with respect to their body of professional knowledge and practice (Friedman and Phillips, 2004: 363) and the dynamically changing traditions of professionalism (Friedman et al., 2008). This is further compounded by a myriad of interchangeable terms: *continuing (professional) education, CPD and lifelong learning*, each of which has a variety of conflicting definitions. The one distinguishing feature that appears to separate the terms hinges on the value attributed to particular learning activities with formal academic learning being favoured particularly as it carries more weight and credibility than informal and work-based learning.

Although definitions of CPD vary they share some common fundamental features in that they should be continuous, profession focused and broad based (Kennie, 1998), and encompass the following principles:

- Be patient centred.
- Responsibility for the management of learning lies with the individual practitioner.
- Involve participation on behalf of the relevant stakeholders (practitioner/organization/education provider/professional regulator).
- Educationally effective.
- Learning needs should be clearly stated and reflect the wider objectives of the organization locally and nationally.

- Enhance the knowledge and skills of the practitioner.
- Involve the application of evidence-based research and practice.
- Learning should be an integral part of everyday working practice rather than seen as a burden.

The final principle is an important one and reiterates how ODPs should view CPD. It should not be about doing just enough to meet the requirements of registration, nor should it be left to the last minute. It should, be as Kennie states, a continuous and ongoing process that becomes embedded in our everyday practices and is therefore something to be embraced as the benefits of engaging in learning can be bountiful and productive.

## Exploring the benefits of CPD

So what are the advantages or benefits of engaging in CPD? Just as there endures differing views and definitions of CPD, the benefits of engaging in learning are wider reaching: with the ODP, the organization, the professional body, and most importantly the patients are all beneficiaries of learning and development.

An individual ODP each has their own perceptions of what CPD can 'do' for us and the reasons for undertaking particular learning activities. These may be linked to immediate short-term goals such as training on new equipment, or updating knowledge around current policies. Longer-term professional development goals may include career-oriented needs such as promotion, extended roles or advanced practitioner roles. Within our own professional context engagement in CPD should be of benefit to us in terms of own development but equally focused and directed towards caring for our patients. Furthermore, it serves to ensure that we carry out our roles and responsibilities safely and effectively as defined by our scope of practice.

### Stop and think

Think about a recent learning activity you have undertaken.

What was its purpose? What have you learned from it? And in what way has it benefited you?

In what way has your learning benefited your patient?

Sadler-Smith et al. (2000) identify three main reasons for undertaking CPD – mobility, maintenance and survival. Evidence from across the literature indicates similar motives: personal development, career/job satisfaction/increased confidence in carrying out our various roles and an updating of knowledge and skills (Murphy et al., 2006). For some practitioners CPD is synonymous with *credentialism* (Morgan et al., 2008), where obtaining academic qualifications provides a 'simple selection for recruitment and promotion' (Hewison et al., 2000: 270). Conversely, some ODPs may view CPD as a necessary evil 'to prevent them going backwards . . . rather than to advance themselves' (Murphy et al., 2006: 378) or through 'fear of being overtaken by less experienced but more academically qualified staff' (Dowswell et al., 1997: 546). Rothwell and Arnold (2005) focus on professional dimensions citing 'avoiding one's license to practice' and 'affirming the individual as a good professional' (Rothwell and Arnold 2005: 29), which are equally valid reasons for undertaking learning.

Moving away from learning simply as a means for personal gain such as promotion and maintaining registration, regular engagement in CPD activities is acknowledged as having a number of further benefits. It can help build confidence within your roles and increases your credibility as a registered ODP as well as developing coping mechanisms to manage the changing environment and updating your skill set. Regular reviews of learning and reflection highlight gaps in learning, knowledge and experience that enables you to take responsibility for developing a learning structure. Linking learning to your annual appraisal enables you to measure your achievements as an individual. Learning within your practice area and alongside colleagues promotes better staff morale, develops a motivated workforce that ultimately results in enhancing patient care. As organizations have shifted responsibility for learning onto the individual practitioner, the ability of the individual to take that responsibility and plan their own professional development is seen as a significant strength. Having a learning framework furthermore aids the organization in planning the learning needs of the workforce that align with wider business objectives and helps in linking theory to practice.

Motivation almost certainly plays a part in our pursuit of learning. According to Smith and Spurling (2005) motivation is a multifaceted concept and loosely defined as 'the personal experience of keenness for pursuing an intended action or goal' (Smith and Spurling 2005: 2). A number of factors are recognized as being responsible for directing individual's pursuit of an intended goal. McGivney (1990) cites three motivating factors that may influence an ODP's pursuit of a particular learning activity: extrinsic, intrinsic and social. Extrinsic factors are varied within the healthcare sector but are mainly driven by government policies and dictates that determine service needs, local initiatives and target setting. Extrinsic factors that directly influence the individual primarily relate to incentives, rewards or positive re-enforcement for engaging in a particular practice or goal. Within the context of learning, external factors such as meeting organizational requirements as part of our employment status, such as completion of statutory and mandatory training, and maintaining competence to practice within our professional remit, provide external motivation.

Intrinsic factors derive from an internal desire and are considered stronger and more enduring than extrinsic factors (Rogers, 2002: 95). Intrinsic factors emanate from the individual through a need to succeed or survive (Maslow, 1954). These are often related to our professional identity or a sense of belonging to a particular group as a way of establishing ourselves among our peers and colleagues. This in itself echoes the strong relationship that learning and CPD have for professionals. Motivation is further governed by the expectancy of rewards or success that could include job satisfaction, benefiting patient care or promotion.

**Stop and think**

What motivates you in your choice of learning activities?

## Planning and managing CPD

How do we plan and manage our CPD? According to Megginson and Whittaker (2007) successful learning is founded on a mutual relationship between employer and employee where both parties benefit from the learning undertaken. The ODP is proactive in determining their own learning needs, is empowered by the process and learning becomes 'an integral part of all work activity' (Megginson and Whittaker, 2007: 5). Field (2006: 206) extends this view arguing in favour of a 'balance of responsibilities between individuals, employers and state'.

The majority of our learning activities are determined through internal processes, although some learning can be *ad hoc*. However, the appraisal system or personal development plan is often the best way to plan your learning needs for the coming 12 months. This process should involve a discussion with your line manager (or someone who is in a suitable position to advise and direct your goals) who may make suggestions with regard to your development and these may often be reflections of wider organizational strategies. The process can be beneficial for all grades of staff in reviewing their current role/responsibilities/practice performance including a view to future requirements. It can be a useful tool in looking at you as a whole as well as serving to highlight any areas for future personal development. It can also help you focus on the next 12 months – what is going to change such as service delivery changes, and the introduction of new services that may require further training for all staff. Use it as a tool to help you.

You may already have a clear plan of the learning activities you wish to access. You may be considering promotion and wanting to know what is required of you to be eligible to apply. You may want support in extending your scope of practice through applying for advanced roles, or taking on a specialist lead role within your specific area of practice. With regard to applying for study leave or funding, it may be beneficial to consult your local education and training policy as each organization will have different processes. This may also provide an insight into the organization's education strategy. There is a tendency for learning activities to be prioritized according to wider organizational objectives. Your local training and education policy should clearly indicate which learning activities are considered priority and may therefore be better supported in terms of financial support or study time.

Although the appraisal process may at times appear time consuming and perhaps often unfulfilled, it can be a valuable exercise as it helps to contribute towards developing the organization's training needs analysis. This in turn feeds into wider stakeholders and commissioning processes for learning activities either locally/in-house or in partnership with local HEI and the commissioners of education.

## Which forms of learning constitute CPD?

A much-held myth is that CPD is all about formal, academic study. This is not the case. Learning under the CPD umbrella and advocated by the HCPC in its earlier definition takes an inclusive approach that serves to incorporate formal, informal, work-based and incidental learning. Within their guide to CPD the HCPC provide a comprehensive but not prescriptive list of learning activities that offers guidance and ideas under five headings: work-based learning, professional activity, formal/educational, self-directed learning and other. From a practitioner perspective, and in accordance with the HCPC requirements of CPD, it is considered good practice to have a broad spread of learning activities.

In adopting a 'context-driven' and outcomes-based approach to CPD, the HCPC acknowledges that ODPs' engagement in learning activities are determined by a number of issues. ODPs' roles, responsibilities and practice interests vary; learning opportunities will differ between organizations, as too will the learning styles and preferences of individual practitioners. Furthermore, it is important to remember that ODPs' learning needs will vary depending on how long they have been qualified and the position they hold within their department – the learning needs of a newly qualified ODP will differ considerably from a senior practitioner with management responsibilities. In addition, engagement in particular learning activities will be influenced by your practice context, your scope of practice as well as wider organizational service needs. An ODP practising within the anaesthetic remit will have different learning needs to one who practises primarily as a surgical practitioner, and will further differ from those ODPs who practise outside of the normal theatre environment.

### Stop and think

You may be considering promotion or know of forthcoming developmental opportunities.

Are you in a position to apply for these opportunities?

What do you need to be doing to enable you to apply and be successful?

## Formal learning

Merriam et al. (2007) define formal learning as 'highly institutionalized, bureaucratic, curriculum driven and formally recognized with grades, diplomas and certificates' (Merriam et al., 2007: 29). This definition epitomizes the generally held view of both learning and education that takes place within specific buildings or institutions, at specific times during a learner's lifetime and between distinctive parties; that of teachers educating and student's being educated (Curtis and Pettigrew, 2010: 154).

As previously stated, CPD is not all about formal/academic learning, although gaining a degree is held in high regard particularly within the healthcare sector as it is considered more effective in delivering patient care (Davey and Robinson, 2002). For some ODPs embarking on a degree pathway may be a personal goal, a requirement of your own career development, as well as an essential element of a senior theatre practitioner. Some ODPs may wish to top up their current qualification after a suitable period post-qualification while the enthusiasm for formal/academic learning is still present. For those ODPs who may not be motivated or disposed towards completing a full degree pathway, there are other options available within this category. As part of your personal and professional development you may be required to undertake the mentorship programme; for some senior practitioner roles this is an essential criterion and will be stipulated within your job description. This standalone module enables you to teach and assess student ODPs during their clinical placements in accordance with the guidelines set out by CODP (2009). Involvement in supporting students also constitutes professional activity under the HCPC's list of CPD activities. You may even consider developing your skills within the education field and enrolling on a specific teacher-training module. Embarking on this specific module may also provide the incentive to continue studying at this level.

Neither is formal learning all about obtaining a degree or undertaking degree-level programmes. Your own organization may run recognized in-house formal courses such as immediate and advanced life support, or management and leadership programmes particularly for newly promoted staff. Your own personal interests may also lead you to take on additional link roles such as infection control, health and safety or manual handling trainer. Have you considered becoming a cascade trainer for medical equipment? These lead roles are often supported and run by your organization but can be supplemented by formal programmes delivered by external providers.

## Work-based learning activities

Some ODPs may not be disposed towards formal learning and prefer the practical, hands-on and work-based learning activities that are directly applicable to their clinical roles. Within the literature, workplace learning usually comes under the informal learning umbrella due to its unstructured nature. And as such it often receives less attention and is perceived as having less credibility than learning associated with formal qualification-conferring. *But work-based learning is an extremely valuable, easily accessible and beneficial form of learning that cannot be underestimated.*

Stephen Billett is a champion of work-based learning and campaigns towards establishing work-based learning as a form of learning in its own right. He emphasizes the value and importance of 'interactions with human partners and non-human artefacts that contribute to an individual's capacity to perform' (Billett, 2004: 316). Our own workplace and through participating in our day-to-day practices can create a wealth of learning opportunities. Although no formal curriculum exists within this learning strategy, the repetitive and ritualistic nature of work practices develops its own evolving and continuous curriculum. Every day can present new and exciting challenges and opportunities for learning – new equipment, new techniques and new procedures provide a richness of new knowledge and skills. Our current and expanding roles can often bring us into contact with other healthcare practitioners who provide opportunities for learning, sharing new ideas and best practices. As a consequence our immediate workplace assumes a more prominent position as a learning environment. As Eraut points out in his exploration of professional knowledge and competence 'professionals continually learn on the job because their work entails engagement in a succession of cases, problems or projects which they have to learn about' (Eraut, 2006: 10). Have you encountered a new surgical procedure, anaesthetic technique, a new piece of medical equipment or drug recently? What impact has this had on your practice? What have you learned from it?

It is likely that you may supervise other staff and students accessing your department, as well as teaching and supporting them you might also learn from them. The wealth of knowledge held within the workplace, particularly with respect to the more experienced practitioners, provides opportunities for discussion, clinical supervision, shadowing, mentoring, networking and cascade learning that are all recognized as valued CPD activities (HCPC, 2012b). The merits of work-based learning rests in its direct applicability to everyday practice whereby highly specific, as well as transferable knowledge and skills, are developed and applied directly to patient care.

In terms of self-directed learning, this can take different directions and is a valuable learning activity. How many journals do you see lying around in the coffee room or left in theatre? Have you picked them up and read some of the articles? What did you think of the articles? Have you discussed changes in practice with colleagues? Have you been prompted to look up a new or unfamiliar procedure on the Internet? Has one of your students asked you a question that you cannot answer? Reflective practice is another valuable learning activity, and one that is discussed in depth in Chapter 8.

When learning becomes part of our everyday practice, it helps contribute to our own motivation, interest and sustainability of engagement in learning practices. Rather than waiting for learning opportunities to come to you, you may become motivated to actively seek out or set up learning activities within your own department such as journal clubs, case study presentations, departmental meetings and clinical audit. Have you considered writing an article for a professional journal? Have you reported back on any training you have recently undertaken or been involved in?

## CPD for the newly qualified ODP

It is recognized that the transition from student ODP to newly qualified practitioner can be daunting and challenging. Support and guidance during the first six to twelve months can be of benefit, and many Trusts have adopted a preceptorship framework for this purpose (DH, 2008). This programme of support and study, which is aimed towards all newly qualified (non-medical) healthcare professionals, aims to enhance the competence and confidence of registered practitioners with the intention of being:

A foundation period of preceptorship for practitioners at the start of their careers will help them begin the journey from novice to expert. This will enable them to apply knowledge, skills and competences acquired as students, into their area of practice, laying a solid foundation for life-long learning.

(DH 2008: 4)

A possible pathway for a newly qualified ODP during their first 12 months could include:

- trust/local induction/preceptorship programme;
- statutory and mandatory training;
- specialty specific learning;
- rotation of anaesthesia, surgery and post anaesthetic care;
- medical devices training;
- blood transfusion – including cell salvage;
- immediate/advanced life support;
- cannulation/venepuncture/catheterization;
- supporting healthcare students in practice that may include formal mentorship training;
- appraisal and planning learning for the next 12 months.

The above list is not meant to be prescriptive but offers some possible suggestions for development during the first year as a newly qualified ODP and leading into the two-year audit period for registration. Being a newly qualified ODP does not mean that you are not already thinking ahead. It is important to remember, however, that your CPD particularly during your first 12 months (and indeed during your later career) will depend on your role and areas of practice as well as the requirements of your department and organization.

So what about someone who has been qualified a few years? As your career progresses your CPD requirements will reflect your developing roles, responsibilities, experiences and interests. How can you continue to meet your professional responsibilities? Here are some possible suggestions:

- completion of statutory and mandatory training;
- reflection in and on practice;
- rotation to various specialisms to update/enhance skills;
- shadowing/secondment;
- deputizing for senior staff/colleagues;
- clinical supervision;
- link person for infection control/health and safety/diabetes;
- specialist interest area or lead practitioner;
- cascade trainer for medical equipment;
- mentoring and teaching of students;
- preceptor for newly qualified staff;
- undertake surgical first assistant or surgical care practitioner education;
- undertake appraisals for 'junior' staff;
- undertake clinical audit;
- undertake further formal academic awards;
- implement or change aspects of practice;
- leadership/management experience/responsibilities;
- reading/reviewing journal articles.

## CPD and the re-registration process

As you are aware, in order to continue to practise and use the protected title of ODP, we are required to renew our registration every two years. This process helps the HCPC demonstrate that their registrants are maintaining their competence, knowledge and skills to practise and meeting their standards.

The HCPC randomly selects a percentage of the ODP registrants to submit their CPD profile detailing their learning activities over the previous two years. The HCPC does state that only those registrants who have been on the register for a full two years are eligible for selection for audit (HCPC, 2012c). This allows those individuals sufficient time to undertake CPD and meet the specific requirements of the HCPC.

The HCPC *Standards of Continuing Professional Development* (HCPC, 2012b) require you to:

1. Maintain an accurate and up-to-date record of your CPD activities.
2. Demonstrate that your CPD activities are a mixture of learning activities relevant to your current and future practice.
3. Ensure that your CPD contributes to the quality of your practice and service delivery.
4. Ensure that the CPD activities benefit the service user.
5. Upon request, present your written profile, complete with supporting evidence explaining how you meet the standards.

## What if I am selected to submit my CPD profile?

So, what if I am selected for audit by the HCPC? First of all, *do not panic*! The HCPC website has all the support information you need to help you complete your continuing professional development profile (www.hcpc-uk.org).

**Stop and think**

If you were selected to submit your CPD profile today how confident are you in meeting the standards?

Make a list of the learning activities you have done over the last three months?

Do you have any evidence to support your learning?

Second, you need to have kept a good record of the learning activities you have undertaken within the specified time period. It is important to remember that keeping a learning log, writing things down and recording your thoughts about your learning and experiences is an essential part of undertaking CPD. We all have different ways of keeping these records; some of us keep a diary of the particular operating lists we do/procedures we have scrubbed for/any incidental or work-based learning activities we have engaged in. You may keep a portfolio of your training and development complete with any certificates of in-house learning you may have completed. One of my colleagues admits to keeping her evidence in a shoe box under her bed! Your line manager or education lead should also have a record of your ongoing training within your department, particularly statutory and mandatory training, which is usually kept for audit purposes. Remember – certificates of attendance are valuable evidence but what is more important is what have you learned from the study/ teaching session? How does it relate to your practice?

Third, however you choose to keep your record of learning activities, it is imperative that they are up to date and can be submitted as evidence if you are selected by the HCPC to do so. Consider it good practice to update your CPD records on a regular basis – weekly or monthly – and do not leave it to the last minute and find yourself scrambling around for certificates or evidence of learning you have undertaken. Personally, I use a mixture of methods for recording my learning: I have a diary for recording any day-to-day activities, a portfolio of training certificates and I have recently started entering my learning activities onto the electronic CPD profile template downloaded from the HCPC website. So, if I am selected by the HCPC for audit I am at least part-way there, and meeting Standards One and Five for CPD.

The requirements for submitting your profile are:

- A summary of your current practice area (maximum 500 words) – this should describe your role and the type of work you undertake, whether you practise primarily within anaesthetics/surgery or recovery or you regularly rotate between the three areas of perioperative practice. Your job description may help you with these aspects. You may rotate between particular specialties or be highly specialized within one area. Who do you communicate with on a daily basis? Do you work in a day-case surgical unit or a large acute Trust with trauma centre status? Perhaps you practise in a non-traditional area such as sterile services or on the transplant team?
- A personal statement (maximum 1,500 words) – select a number of CPD activities (between three and 5) you have undertaken during the specified time period. To fulfil the requirements for profile submission and meet Standard Two, they must be a mixture of learning activities that reflect your current practice and future intentions. Once you have selected your CPD activities that best

reflect your own personal learning during the specified time period ask yourself the following questions that will help you achieve Standards Three and Four:

**Stop and think**

How has your learning benefited and improved the quality of your practice?

How has your learning benefited the patient and wider service user?

How does your learning enable you to practise safely and effectively?

How does your CPD relate to your changing work practices?

## Barriers to learning

The current difficulties being experienced within the NHS, particularly the financial situation has served to create a less than ideal environment for engaging in CPD. Research indicates that there are a number of barriers towards engaging in CPD including a lack of time coupled with an increased workload (Sturrock and Lennie, 2009), lack of understanding of CPD issues (Bell et al., 2001), shortage of staff and lack of management support (Gould et al., 2007). We have all probably experienced these issues at some point and find it extremely frustrating especially as other healthcare professionals receive 'protected learning time' such as doctors and dentists. So how can we keep up to date with our continuing professional responsibilities and ensure that our knowledge, skills and performance are of a high quality while overcoming these barriers to learning? Here are some suggestions and examples of possible CPD activities:

- Be prepared to do some CPD in your own time. You may be able to claim the time in lieu.
- Utilize your time effectively. Do you have theatre downtime/audit meetings? Do you regularly attend department meetings or undertake a form of clinical supervision?
- If you have the opportunity have you considered setting up and running training or study days yourself?
- Be flexible – if you are funded for a course you may be required to study in your own time. Conversely, you may be offered study time if you fund/part-fund study. This will depend on you organization's policy.
- Online or e-learning modules are widely available. Some HEIs deliver the mentorship programme online/distance. The Blood Transfusion Service has good e-learning packages particularly on cell salvage.
- Medical companies and representatives are often willing to give up their time to deliver specific training sessions. Some have teaching/learning packages.
- What is available in your department? Some medical staff may be willing to do some teaching/training sessions as part of their own development.

## Conclusion

The aim of this chapter was to explore the concepts and practices of CPD within the specific context of operating department practice. Mandatory CPD is a relatively new concept for many of us but one that has become an integral aspect of our professional identity and professional practice. But there is flexibility and personal choice in how we learn and the types of learning we engage in – remember that the learning you undertake should be relevant to your current or future role, be of benefit to your practice, your patients and service user.

## Key points

- CPD is an essential component of operating department practice and should be integral to every ODP's role.
- CPD serves to benefit the learner, the organization and most importantly the patient.
- CPD can be achieved by a number of methods and ODPs should undertake a number of different activities.
- ODPs must be able to submit evidence of their CPD if selected for audit by the HCPC in the advised format.

## References and further reading

Bell, H.M., Maguire, T.A., Adair, C.G. and McGartland, L.F. (2001) 'Perceptions of CPD within the pharmacy profession', *International Journal of Pharmacy Practice*, 9 (S1): 55.

Biggs, J. and Tang, C. (2011) *Teaching for Quality Learning at University* (4th edn). Maidenhead: Open University Press.

Billett, S. (2004) 'Workplace participatory practices: conceptualising workplaces as learning environments', *Journal of Workplace Learning*, 16 (6): 312–24.

*British Journal of Obstetrics and Gynaecology: An International Journal of Obstetrics and Gynaecology* (2011) Special Issue. 'Saving mother's lives: reviewing maternal deaths to make motherhood safer: 2006-2008'. The Eighth Report of the Confidential Enquiries into Maternal Deaths in the United Kingdom, 118 (S1): 1–203.

College of Operating Department Practitioners (CODP) (2009) *Standards, Recommendations and Guidance for Mentors and Practice Placements: Supporting Pre-registration Education in Operating Department Practice Provision*. London: CODP.

College of Operating Department Practitioners (CODP) (2010) Discussion paper, 'Framing the future role and function of Operating Department Practitioners'. London: CODP.

College of Operating Department Practitioners (CODP) (2012) 'Notice of withdrawal of the pre-registration DipHE Operating Department Practice Curriculum, *Technic*, 3 (6): 7.

Curtis, W. and Pettigrew, A. (2010) *Education Studies: Reflective Reader*. Exeter: Learning Matters.

Davey, B. and Robinson, S. (2002) 'Taking a degree after qualifying as a registered general nurse: constraints and effects', *Nurse Education Today*, 22: 624–32.

Department of Health (DH) (2001) *Bristol Royal Infirmary Final Report*. London: DH.

Department of Health (DH) (2003) *Modernising Medical Careers: The Response of Four UK Health Ministers to the Consultation on Unfinished Business: Proposals for Reform*. London: DH.

Department of Health (DH) (2004) *Learning for Delivery: Making Connections between Post Qualification Learning/Continuing Professional Development and Service Planning*. London: DH.

Department of Health (DH) (2008) *High Quality Care for All, Next Stage Review: Final Report*. London: DH.

Department of Health (DH) (2009a) *Preceptorship Framework for Newly Qualified Nurses, Midwives and Allied Health Professionals*. London: DH.

Department of Health (DH) (2009b) *European Working Time Directive: UK Notification of Derogation for Doctors in Training*. Available online at http://webarchive.nationalarchives.gov.uk/+/www.dh.gov.uk/en/publicationsandstatistics/publications/publicationspolicyandguidance/dh_093940 (accessed 10 November 2013).

Department of Health (DH) (2010) *NHS Constitution: The NHS Belongs to Us All*. Available online at https://www.gov.uk/government/publications/the-nhs-constitution-for-england (accessed 10 November 2013).

Department of Health (DH) (2012) *Liberating the NHS: Developing the Healthcare Workforce. From Design to Delivery*. London: DH.

Dowswell, T., Hewison, J. and Millare, B. (1997) 'Joining the learning society and working in the NHS: some issues', *Journal of Education Policy*, 12 (6): 539–50.

Earley, P. and Bubb, S. (2007) *Leading and Managing Continuing Professional Development: Developing People, Developing Schools*. London: Paul Chapman Publishing.

Ellis, R. (1998) *Professional Competence and Quality Assurance in the Caring Professions*. London: Chapman and Hall.

Eraut, M. (2006) *Developing Professional Knowledge and Competence*. London: Falmer Press.

Field, J. (2006) *Lifelong Learning and the New Educational Order*. Stoke-on-Trent: Trentham Books.

Francis Report (2013) *Report of the Mid Staffordshire NHS Foundation Trust Public Enquiry Executive Summary*. London: Stationery Office.

Friedman, A. and Phillips, P. (2004) 'Continuing professional development: developing a vision', *Journal of Education and Work*, 17 (3): 361–76.

Friedman, A., William, C., Hopkins, S. and Jackson, L. (2008) *Linking Professional Associations with Higher Education Institutions (HEIs) in Relation to the Provision of Continuing Professional Development*. Bristol: Professional Associations Research Network.

Gallagher, L. (2007) 'Continuing education in nursing: a concept analysis', *Nurse Education Today*, 27: 466–73.

Gardner, R. (1978) *Policy on Continuing Education: A Report with Recommendations for Action*. York: University of York.

Gould, D., Drey, N. and Berridge, E. (2007) 'Nurses' experiences of continuing professional development', *Nurse Education Today*, 27: 602–09.

Handy, C. (1993) *Understanding Organisations*. London: Penguin.

Health and Care Professions Council (HCPC) (2004) *Continuing Professional Development – Consultation Paper*. London: HCPC.

Health and Care Professions Council (HCPC) (2012a) *The Standards of Conduct, Performance and Ethics*. London: HCPC.

Health and Care Professions Council (HCPC) (2012b) *Your Guide to our Standards of Continuing Professional Development*. London: HCPC.

Health and Care Professions Council (HCPC) (2012c) *Continuing Professional Development and your Registration*. London: HCPC.

Health and Care Professional Council (HCPC) (2012d) *How to Complete your Continuing Professional Development Profile*. London: HCPC.

Health and Care Professions Council (HCPC) (2014) *Standards of Proficiency: Operating Department Practitioners*. London: HCPC.

Hewison, J., Dowswell, T. and Millar, B. (2000) 'Changing patterns of training provision in the National Health Service: an overview', in Coffield, F (ed.) *Differing Visions of a Learning Society: Research Findings Volume 1*. Bristol: The Policy Press.

James, N. (2007) 'The learning trajectories of "old-timers": academic identities and communities of practice in higher education', in Hughes, J., Jewson, N. and Unwin, L. (eds) *Communities of Practice: Critical Perspectives*. Oxford: Routledge.

Jarvis, P. (2007) *Adult Education and Lifelong Learning* (3rd edn). London: Routledge Falmer.

Kennie, T.J.M. (1998) 'The growing importance of CPD', *Continuing Professional Development*, 1: 160–69.

Longworth, N. (2003) *Lifelong Learning in Action: Transforming Education in the 21st Century*. London: Routledge Falmer.

Maben, J., Latter, S. and Macleod Clark, J. (2006) 'The theory-practice gap: impact of professional-bureaucratic work conflict on newly-qualified nurses', *Journal of Advanced Nursing*, 55 (4): 465–77.

Maslow, A. (1954) *Motivation and Personality*. New York: Harper.

McGivney, V. (1990) *Education's for Other People: Access to Education for Non-Participant Adults*. Leicester: National Institute of Adult Continuing Education.

Megginson, D. and Whittaker, V. (2007) *Continuing Professional Development*. London: Chartered Institute of Personnel and Development.

Merriam, S., Caffarella, R. and Baumgartner, L. (2007) *Learning in Adulthood: A Comprehensive Guide* (3rd edn). New York: John Wiley & Sons, Inc.

Morgan, A., Cullinane, J. and Pye. M. (2008) 'Continuing professional development: rhetoric and practice in the NHS', *Journal of Education and Work*, 21 (3): 233–48.

Murphy, C., Cross, C. and McGuire, D. (2006) 'The motivation of nurses to participate in continuing professional education', *Journal of European Industrial Training*, 30 (5): 365–84.

National Patient Safety Agency (NPSA) (2004) *Seven Steps to Patient Safety: An Overview Guide for Staff*. London: NPSA.

Patient Safety First (2010) *Implementing Human Factors in Healthcare: 'How to' Guide*. Available online at www.patientsafetyfirst.nhs.uk

Rogers, A. (2002) *Teaching Adults* (3rd edn). Maidenhead: Open University Press.

Roscoe, J. (2002) 'Continuing professional development in higher education', *Human Resource Development International*, 5 (1): 3–9.

Rothwell, A. and Arnold, J. (2005) 'How HR professionals rate "continuing professional development"', *Human Resource Management Journal*, 15 (3): 18–32.

Sadler-Smith, E., Allinson, C.W. and Hayes, J. (2000) 'Learning preferences and cognitive style: some implications for continuing professional development', *Management Learning*, 31 (2): 239–56.

Schön, D.A. (1983) *The Reflective Practitioner. How Professionals Think in Action*. Farnham: Ashgate Publishing Limited.

Smith, J. and Spurling A. (2005) *Understanding Motivation for Lifelong Learning*. London: Campaign for Learning.

Sturrock, J.B.E. and Lennie, S.C. (2009) 'Compulsory continuing professional development: a questionnaire-based survey of the UK dietetic profession', *Journal of Human Nutrition and Dietetics*, 22: 12–20.

Watkins, J. (1999) 'UK professional associations and continuing professional development: a new direction', *International Journal of Lifelong Learning*, 18 (1): 61–75.

# Index

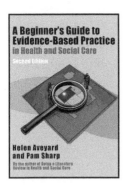

## BEGINNER'S GUIDE TO EVIDENCE-BASED PRACTICE IN HEALTH AND SOCIAL CARE

Second Edition

Helen Aveyard and Pam Sharp

9780335246724 (Paperback)
April 2013

eBook also available

**Have you heard of 'evidence based practice' but don't know what it means?
Are you having trouble relating evidence to your practice?**

This is **the** book for anyone who has ever wondered what evidence based practice is or how to relate it to practice. Fully updated in this brand new edition, this book is simple and easy to understand – and designed to help those new to the topic to apply the concept to their practice and learning with ease.

**Key features:**

- Additional material on literature reviews and searching for literature
- Even more examples for health and social care practice
- Extra material on qualitative research and evidence based practice
- Expanded section on hierarchies of evidence and how to use them

www.openup.co.uk

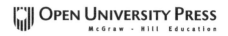

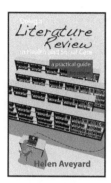

**Doing a Literature Review in Health and Social Care**
A Practical Guide
Third Edition

Helen Aveyard

9780335263073 (Paperback)
January 2014

eBook also available

This bestselling book is a step-by-step guide to doing a literature review in health and social care. It is vital reading for all those undertaking their undergraduate or postgraduate dissertation or any research module which involves a literature review. The book provides a practical guide to doing a literature review from start to finish.

**Key features:**

- Even more examples of real life research scenarios
- More emphasis on how to ask the right question
- New and updated advice on following a clear search strategy

www.openup.co.uk

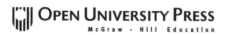 OPEN UNIVERSITY PRESS
McGraw · Hill Education

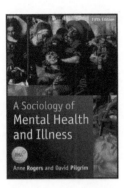

**A SOCIOLOGY OF MENTAL HEALTH AND ILLNESS**
Fifth Edition

Anne Rogers and David Pilgrim

9780335262762 (Paperback)
May 2014

eBook also available

How do we understand mental health problems in their social context?
   A former BMA Medical Book of the Year award winner, this book provides a sociological analysis of major areas of mental health and illness. The book considers contemporary and historical aspects of sociology, social psychiatry, policy and therapeutic law to help students develop an in-depth and critical approach to this complex subject.

**Key features:**

- Brand new chapter on prisons, criminal justice and mental health
- Expanded coverage of stigma, class and social networks
- Updated material on the Mental Capacity Act, Mental Health Act and the Deprivation of Liberty

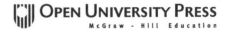

www.openup.co.uk